The Commonsense Guide to Good Eating

By

Barbara E. Echols,
Director of Office of Grants and Contracts,
Duke University Medical Center

Jay M. Arena, M.D.,
Professor of Pediatrics,
Duke University Medical Center

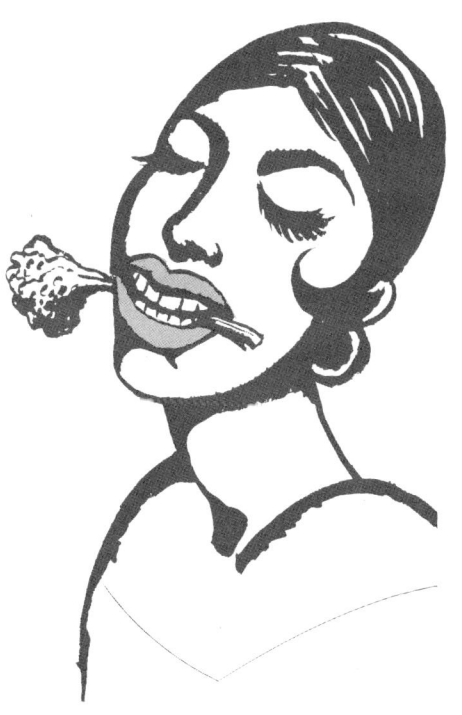

BARRON'S / WOODBURY, NEW YORK

©Copyright 1978 by Barron's Educational Series, Inc.

All rights reserved.
No part of this book may be reproduced
in any form, by photostat, microfilm, xerography,
or any other means, or incorporated into any
information retrieval system, electronic or
mechanical, without the written permission
of the copyright owner.

All inquiries should be addressed to:
Barron's Educational Series, Inc.
113 Crossways Park Drive
Woodbury, New York 11797

Library of Congress Catalog Card No. 77-862

International Standard Book No. 0-8120-0791-3

Library of Congress Cataloging in Publication Data
Echols, Barbara E
The Commonsense Guide to Good Eating
Bibliography: p. 171
  1. Nutrition. 2. Diet. I. Arena, Jay M.,
joint author. II. Title.
RA784.E25   613.2   77-862
ISBN 0-8120-0791-3

PRINTED IN THE UNITED STATES OF AMERICA

Contents

v   *Foreword by William J. Darby, President, The Nutrition Foundation, Inc.*

vii   *Preface*

xi   *Introduction: Why are Americans flunking "food"?*

1   *One/Your Body—What Are You Doing To It?*
Seven questions to help you assess your nutritional knowledge

5   *Two/Food, Glorious Food*
A discussion of your nutrient requirements

19   *Three/Food for Thought*
Five goals, plus information about eating habits

29   *Four/Vegetarianism—Fad or "A Different Way"?*
The problems and the benefits

35   *Five/What About Health Foods?*
The real concerns, plus some questions and answers

43   *Six/Your Weight—Good or Bad?*
Nine questions and answers about your weight

53   *Seven/I'm Overweight! Now What?*
Causes and treatment, plus some questions and answers

The Commonsense Guide to Good Eating

69 *Eight/At the Store and In Your Kitchen*
Practicing what we've preached!

75 *Nine/How to Plan Your Meals Without Counting Calories*
A food exchange program plus diet plans from 800 to 3000 calories for those who want to regulate their weight and improve their nutrient intake

91 *Ten/Atherosclerosis—Prevention Begins at an Early Age*
Information and recommendations about a disease process that probably begins in childhood

101 *Eleven/Diabetes*
Causes and treatment plus some questions and answers

107 *Twelve/Special Dietary Problems*
Food sensitivities, acne, dental health, pregnancy, physical training programs, and some problems of the poor and the elderly

117 *Thirteen/Food Poisoning*
Words of warning

131 *Appendix I   Recipes: Main meals which convert to great lunchbox ideas*

147 *Appendix II The Whys and Wherefores of Vitamins and Minerals*

169 *Notes*

171 *Bibliography*

Foreword

Issues surrounding food and nutrition are widely debated, in large part because of limited knowledge and understanding of many concerning simple fundamental facts about foods and the physiology of nutrition. Very few young people today have the opportunity to participate in growing, harvesting, storing or other steps, in producing food. Less than four percent of our population grows the food which feeds us all. People buy their food in various stages of preparation or ready to eat. They have little need to be involved in its production. Knowledge of what is food, therefore, is not developed as it was traditionally when the major food was produced on the farm by the family with all members being involved in its procurement.

For two or more generations food and nutrition have been neglected as subjects in the curriculum of most schools. During this same period, there has been an increasing awareness that our health is dependent upon the nature of the food we eat and our nutritional state. As a result, people widely question whether they are maintaining the best state of nutritional health for themselves and their families.

Writers, entertainers, speakers, promoters, scientists and nonscientists, and even outright charlatans disseminate factual information, false information, truths and half-truths, and frequently leave the interested individual in a state of confused anxiety or with a conviction that has no factual or scientific basis.

The purveyors of "nutrition gospel" make sensational claims that promise health, super prowess in athletics, long life, sexual potency, or offer cures or relief from incurable diseases. Their promises have wide appeal because they promise without reservation or qualification that which people want. This type of writing or message is readily saleable and profitable. The result is a plethora of sensational, often fallacious books about this or that diet which cures or prevents some widely feared condition.

The Commonsense Guide to Good Eating

Sane, balanced discussion that presents the facts concerning food and nutrition without exaggeration is neither sensational nor newsworthy, hence it goes unheralded. These books, however, should be widely read. They are the ones that can contribute to an understanding of foods and nutrition in a manner to promote a lifetime of maximum benefit from good food habits. Such a book, interestingly written, balanced in perspective and based upon scientific understanding, has been prepared by the authors of *The Commonsense Guide to Good Eating.* Those who read this guide will be indebted to Barbara E. Echols and Jay M. Arena, both of Duke University Medical Center.

William J. Darby, M.D., Ph.D.
President, The Nutrition Foundation, Inc.

Preface

One of the issues in contemporary nutrition education today is the role of the media in educating the consumer. The influence of the news media, of the press (books and magazines), and especially of TV, particularly on children, is enormous and oftentimes devastating by its faddist misinformation. There are more commercials altogether, and proportionately more food commercials, on children's television than on adult television—about three-fourths of the estimated 22 commercials an hour that are aimed at children are for edible products. These advertised edible products are on the whole nutritionally poor and, unfortunately, children—since they are in the process of establishing food preferences and attitudes which may affect their eating habits for life—are an especially vulnerable audience. The American public is looking for nutritional information that is more than a current fad. They are trying to develop new eating patterns with very little available practical and sensible instruction and no family tradition to help them.

Traditionally, nutrition education has been offered as a part of home economics or has been attached to subjects such as biology or physical education. In most instances, this subject has not been offered at all. Even when available, nutrition education has consistently suffered from the major defect of lack of involvement of the intended audience in the planning of the program and, hence, lack of relevant subject matter and educational materials.

As a consequence, we see programs focused on the three-meals-a-day, four-basic-food-groups pattern with little attention paid to outside influences, individual preferences and concerns, or ethical and economic considerations. For example:
- Authoritative manuals abound on the need for vitamins and minerals and their importance in preventing scurvy, rickets, etc. But little is available to the general public citing both sides of the vitamin C megadose controversy.
- Vegetarianism is still often presented as "food fadism," and those concerned

about food additives are viewed as "health food nuts."
- Dieters, like smokers, are told that "motivation" and "will power" are the answers to their dilemma. Little is offered in the way of linking knowledge to practical mechanisms that will enable people to adopt and maintain more healthful habits.

It is not surprising, then, that consumers exhibit a certain wariness when approached with additional information that is "good for them" to know.

In 1974, we went into one of the local high schools with a questionnaire designed to elicit present nutrition knowledge, attitudes, and areas of interest. The results revealed a conspicuous lack of knowledge about the relationship of nutrition to health in general, and about the students' own personal and specific needs. We were not surprised, therefore, to see the number of students who described their weight as other than "desirable," and who stated that they did not know if they were meeting their nutritional requirements.

Next, we assembled a group of student volunteers with which one of us met twice a week at lunchtime. Either the students or we prepared the meal, aiming for variety, nutritional soundness in keeping with our present knowledge about the relationship of food to health, and caloric and cost containment. By mutual agreement, the meals were mostly vegetarian so as not to offend the dietary preferences of some of the students. This latter consideration not only educated our palate—many of us were not familiar with some of the staples which are standard in the vegetarian household—but illustrated the feasibility of obtaining all the essential amino acids without the use of meats.

The students and we started out with the hypothesis that working together, we could design a more meaningful and interesting nutrition curriculum than either of us could alone. We then outlined the following approach:

   1. Identify what aspects of nutrition are felt to be of interest and concern. Without agreement on content, we would be repeating the errors of nonrelevance.

   2. Using people and literature resources, identify and make available the most up-to-date information on each nutrition-related topic that has been identified. This would obviously mean presenting both sides of the coin where controversy exists.

   3. In consultation with an educational psychologist and communications expert, design educational materials and experiences for relating the identified information to an audience of the students' peers. Relevance of the mode of information transfer has been deemed to be every bit as important as the content itself.

Through class discussion and independent consideration, a list of nutrition-related topics was developed. It was interesting to note the number of topics identified as important to the students' concerns that are not usually

Preface

covered in the standard texts used in nutrition education programs for this age group. For example, diet needs and problems of the elderly, how foods affect your emotions, the influence of the food industry on our eating patterns, legislative process involving food safety measures, relative effectiveness of chemical versus natural vitamins and organic versus fertilized food production, percent of filth allowable in foods, practical alternatives for the non-meat-eater, cost reduction, the pregnant teenager, etc.

There was little interest in tackling the vitamins and minerals one by one as it is ususally done. Rather, the emphasis seemed to be on individuals' well-being and the influence of their diet as a whole. The students did keep a food diary which was then analyzed in terms of calories, protein, carbohydrates, fat, vitamins, and minerals so they did have some basis for their evaluation of the adequacy of their diet.

The independent research, the sharing of information, and the involvement in decisions and food preparation all offered the student active involvement in the pursuit of nutrition knowledge. In areas of health education, this approach seems more promising than the more passive lecture-test approach.

After completing their reports on the topics they had identified as relevant, the students assembled the material into a small booklet which was distributed to other students, parents, and community members. At the same time, flyers outlining the project and offering to assist other schools, church groups, and community organizations that were interested in planning a nutrition-related project were also circulated.

The Commonsense Guide to Good Eating is an outgrowth of the above project. It addresses the various topics identified by the students and identifies and discusses the major points of controversy where they exist. Every effort has been made to present concisely the latest information available on the relationship of nutrition to health. This material has been presented honestly, accurately, and succinctly. It is no "big production." It is hoped, however, that this book will be an effective and valuable nutritional publication for everyone.

This book would not have been possible without the cooperation of the Carolina Friends School in Orange County, North Carolina, and a dedicated group of their students. We would, therefore, like to thank, by name, those most responsible for the success of the project that identified so many of the topics included in this book: Don Wells, Connie Toverud, Sallie Bolich, Ann Borden, Barbra Bucci, Wesley Clark, Jody Fein, Patty Freeman, Chris Gwyn, Susan Holley, Mely Hodges, Jake Jacobson, Liz Jones, Annie Kachergis, Amy Katzenmyer, Jim Lauderdale, Annie Lipsitz, Nancy Richmond, Corky Williams.

Nor would our thanks be complete without acknowledging the fine guidance and assistance of Dr. Marjorie Boeck in the design of the initial questionnaire and its evaluation, for her contribution to the overall project, and for her faithful reading and re-reading of this manuscript, providing criticism which strengthened the book without deflating our egoes or enthusiásm. Also our thanks to Dr. Jay Skyler for his meticulous review of the book, for his advice (both medical and philosophical), and for his gentle reminders about the subtleties of the English language.

And to our spouses, our children and their friends, and our office staffs go a special word of thanks for they, too, were our constant guinea pigs on whom we often tried ideas.

Introduction

Why are Americans Flunking "Food"?

The fundamental philosophy of nutrition education is that prevention is preferable to cure. In terms of money, time, quality of life, and human resources it can be shown repeatedly that rehabilitation is more costly than prevention. Efforts to focus on prevention of nutritional ill health rather than solely on crisis intervention are needed.

Although our bodies are not in such delicate balance that we need to constantly monitor our food intake, there are certain groups who are more vulnerable to nutritional deficiencies than others: pregnant women, nursing mothers, infants, preschool children, adolescents, the poor, the elderly—especially those living alone, the chronically ill, and the sedentary. Each of these groups represents a complex series of problems, with nutrition being but one of the many elements involved. In each situation, however, it is possible that improving the state of nutrition may also benefit the other problem areas; the reverse is, of course, also true.

One of the stumbling blocks to a better public understanding of the role that nutrition plays in health maintenance is the lack of a readily identifiable, reliable, national source for "state of the art" information. The public receives little help in dealing with controversial issues such as vitamin megadoses and dietary cholesterol. Rather, they must rely on the authority of whomever is presently in the news. Even assistance in weight control—one of our leading health problems—is often hard to come by and, once again, the public is left to evaluate the safety of ketogenic diets, hypnotic suggestion, ear staples, and a variety of shots and pills.

Common to all the problems discussed in this book is the need to influence the developing food and exercise habits of the young child. Additionally, programs are needed to better educate the public regarding the availability of prenatal clinics and other health services, their right and need to use these facilities, and how to use them effectively. Also, the public and their elected representatives need a clearer picture of the nutritional needs of the country. Health and health insurance providers, public assistance programs, and the food industry all have responsible roles and should stand accountable. Nor can we forgo our worldwide responsibilities. Cattle being slaughtered and discarded while people starve to death is a recklessness and a lack of concern for human life and suffering that is hard to comprehend. One of the consequences of our affluency is a lack of appreciation for just how precious food is to many people.

Specific efforts to provide public education might include the following:

1. The support of legislation aimed at increasing the number of professionals qualified to teach comprehensive health education at the elementary and secondary school level.

2. Development of funding sources for pilot and demonstration projects to: a) reassess health education goals and the relevance of current teaching material and practices to the present and future needs of elementary and secondary school students; and b) develop and disseminate curricular materials.

3. Initiation of school-based programs aimed at weight evaluation and regulation. The magnitude of the obesity problem in children is such that reliance cannot be placed on the individual initiative of parents and children to obtain weight therapy when needed. Furthermore, the cost of such therapy through private medicine is generally too high for all but a limited number of individuals. The public school system, therefore, affords one suitable and logical focus for an attack on the problem of weight control.

Cooperation from the medical community and parents would be necessary to safely assess the individual's health and advisability of participating in such an endeavor. The presence of such a project might make both physicians and parents more alert and sympathetic to the minimally overweight person rather than waiting until they're markedly overweight. An extra few pounds is a lot easier and more satisfactorily dealt with than the burden of twenty or thirty pounds and their attendent illnesses. Preventive rather than curative medicine is urged for other areas of bodily concern—why not for fat control?

4. As the character of the available food supply changes to include increasing reliance on fabricated foods, vending machines, and out-of-home feeding in general, nutrition education efforts directed toward food suppliers will become increasingly important. What is available at school, at work, and in the local drive-in will influence the quality of our diet. The individuals who decide which vending machines to install in a factory or a school, for instance, are important targets for nutrition education.

5. A tremendous amount of money is being spent by food manufacturers for the promotion of their products. Considering the influence that the advertising media have over the public's eating habits, if even a part of this

Introduction

effort were directed at reorienting Americans' tastes, it would be a great contribution to the nation's health. It can be hoped that the food industry and television broadcasting companies will become increasingly concerned about their public role and responsibilities.

    6. Federal regulations require labels to indicate nutritional composition if the foods are enriched or fortified or if a nutritional claim is made for the food. Other foods are not required to be so labeled. Many companies have started voluntarily including this type of information on their products' labels. This trend indicates a definite concern for the health of the American people and should be applauded and further encouraged. An educational program will, however, be required if the public is to understand and make use of this information.

    7. It may be impractical to expect individual restaurants to change their preparation practices or to post the caloric values of their foods, but it is not untoward to expect this of school and office cafeterias. There is much that still isn't known about nutritional needs and the consequences of certain deficiencies and excesses, but that which *is* known shouldn't be so blatantly disregarded by institutions responsible for feeding large segments of our society—especially our children. People deserve sufficient information to know what nutrient choices they are making.

    8. Exercise not only helps ward off obesity but it helps to keep arteries unclogged and increases one's chances of recovery should he or she suffer a heart attack. Unfortunately, however, Americans seem to not only have trouble motivating themselves to exercise, but difficulty in motivating their children as well. By the time the average child starts school, he or she has logged over 4,000 hours in front of the television set! To compound the issue, most physical education programs at school and in the community are aimed at the person who is already in pretty good physical condition. Increased opportunities are needed for obese people or otherwise handicapped people to improve their physical activity pattern. Also, patterns of more individual exercise should be encouraged if a life long pattern of participation is to be encouraged. A tennis partner is a lot easier to locate than enough people for a football or volleyball game. Also, governmental provision of safe bicycle paths or lanes would be a boon not only to health but to the energy crisis as well.

    9. To improve the nutrition of the elderly and to take advantage of the influence they exert over younger members in the family, every effort should be made to update their nutritional information. Again, the data provided should be relevant to their needs. Community programs for the elderly and various hobby clubs are two modes of approach. Contacts with club members representing a younger age group might also get the message carried home to parents and grandparents. Businesses could also probably be persuaded to

offer pre-retirement seminars and discussions for their employees, provided adequate instructional materials and guidance were available.

10. Continued research into the relationship of nutrition to health and illness needs to be conducted. In many cases, this may require stimulating faculty to an awareness and interest in the area. Few medical schools have an organizational cluster identified with nutritional concerns. One obvious problem here is the lack of manpower trained or knowledgeable in the field. New types of training experiences may well be called for.

11. Professionals active in the field of nutrition must take increased responsibility for educating the public at large about their perceived needs and concerns. The number of popular food-related books that are in print and are being purchased clearly attests to the public's concern with its diet. Much of the information published is, without question, incorrect or misleading. Too often, however, knowledgeable people and organizations merely attack these lay-oriented publications, without offering practical advice in their stead. It is little wonder then that the public often views health-related professionals as being in an adversary position and turn instead to the miracle-offerers.

12. Hospitals and extended care facilities offer another possibility for educating the public about nutritional concerns. To be effective, however, the food in these institutions would probably have to become more palatable and responsive to the needs of the individual than just to the masses. Serving the same caloric offering to the 100- and 250-pounder alike doesn't say much for one's awareness of individual needs.

Though reimbursement and evaluation mechanisms are not dealt with in this book, their omission should not be construed as indifference to the problems. By the same token, the difficulties involved in financing and assessing health education endeavors should not keep us from trying to move on with the resources at hand.

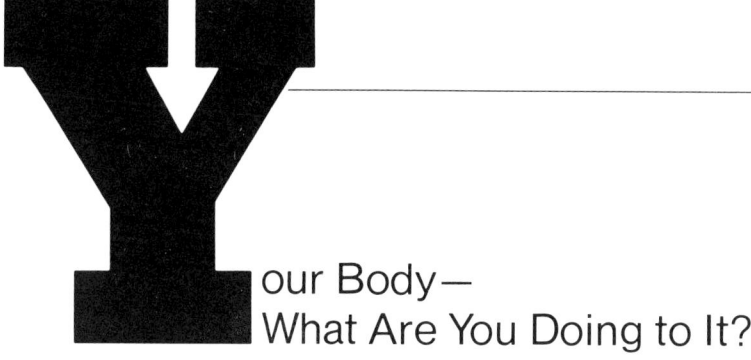
our Body—
What Are You Doing to It?

Seven Questions to Help You Assess Your Nutritional Knowledge

Good nutrition means more than adequate protein and vitamins and minerals. It also means food intake equal to—not more or less than—your body's actual requirements. Both overweight and underweight may signal poor nutrition, as does a diet lacking adequate protein and other nutrients.

Ask yourself the following questions. If you have trouble answering these questions, your nutritional well-being or "know how" may not be as sound as it should be.

Are you eating the right number of calories to maintain your desirable weight and activity level?

If you are consistently consuming more calories than your body needs to meet your physiological requirements, you can expect to continue to gain weight. If you are consistently eating fewer calories than your body requires, you are no doubt underweight or losing weight.

Weight evaluation and regulation is critical to living out your normal life span. The death rate for overweight persons is higher than for those of average weight, and the death rate for persons of average weight is higher than for those of desirable weight. On the other hand, adequate nutrition is vital to the development and maintenance of many body functions necessary for dental health, resistance to infection, freedom from fatigue, and even maintenance of healthy skin and hair. Underweight may signal inadequate nutrient intake.

Are you eating at least three servings each day of meat and/or milk products?

Both meat and milk products are high in protein. If three or more servings each day are coming from these or from other high quality protein sources, your total diet is probably providing fifty to seventy grams of protein. Your protein needs are, thus, being met quite adequately.

Vegetarianism is increasing in this country for a variety of reasons. In many respects, this represents a healthy change. However, since vitamin B_{12} is not found in plants and since most plants are deficient in one or more of the essential amino acids, the vegetarian must have a better knowledge of nutrition than the nonvegetarian to ensure adequate protein (which is made up of amino acids) and vitamin intakes. Neither the B_{12} nor the amino acids is likely to be a problem if eggs, milk, or cheese are routinely included in the diet.

Are more than thirty percent of your calories each day coming from fats?

If so, you ought to consider changing this situation, especially if the fats are mainly "saturated" ones. A thirty to thirty-five percent fat intake is more than adequate to provide the necessary energy, heat, and organ padding required by the body. And don't forget, both milk (unless it is skimmed) and meat are moderately high in fat content — saturated fat at that! Remember, too, the amount of "invisible" fats in food such as nuts and avocadoes.

Excessive amounts of saturated fats may be dangerous to your long-term health. They often contribute to elevated cholesterol levels which, when combined with other undesirable life-style habits such as excessive sugar intake, persistent overweight, tension, cigarette smoking, and inactivity, set the stage for the development of heart disease.

Do you routinely eat eggs?

One egg yolk contains about 275 mg of cholesterol. Add to that the cholesterol in other foods — 30 mg of cholesterol per eight ounces of whole milk, 30 to 35 mg per ounce in hot dogs and hamburgers, etc., and you can see how easy it would be to go over the 300 mg of cholesterol a day that the American Heart Association feels is the maximum intake advisable.

Are you fulfilling your vitamin and mineral requirements?

If your daily diet includes eight ounces of milk; two servings of meat, fish, poultry, or cheese; one citrus fruit; one serving of a dark green or deep yellow vegetable; and one serving of bread or cereal, you are probably meeting your body's requirements.

Periods of physical stress, such as recovery from illness, rapid growth periods, pregnancy, and while nursing a baby place a great burden on the body. Nutritional deficiencies are most injurious during these periods. Extremely low-calorie diets also make it difficult to meet your nutritional needs.

Preliminary studies of the nutritional status of this nation suggest that some segments of our population may have one or more vitamin or mineral deficiencies. If for some reason you can't meet your vitamin and mineral requirements through food selection, take a daily vitamin-mineral supplement. Don't

Your Body—What Are You Doing to It?

take more than is recommended, however. Some vitamins and minerals build up in the body and are extremely dangerous when taken in high doses—so don't overdo it!

Are you a heavy salt user?

If so, you are not doing your blood pressure any favor. A heavy use of salt is associated with an increased likelihood of high blood pressure, causing difficulties for your heart and arteries. Also, excessive intakes of salt can cause the body to retain unusual amounts of water in an attempt to bring the body into chemical balance. The result is increased weight and swelling—most noticeably in the legs and feet—which can be harmful to the kidneys and to the lungs.

If you are the type of person who salts food both as it is cooked and before tasting it, you are a heavy salt user. This does not mean that you should eliminate salt from your diet (though in most cases it is not a necessary dietary additive), but you should at least taste your food before you salt it. You may save yourself future troubles. Remember that there are practically no naturally salt-free foods available.

How much do you know about the "state of the art" concerning the relationship of nutrition to health?

There are many controversial issues involved in the relationship of food to health. In many respects there are more unknowns than knows. Results of laboratory tests involving animals are not necessarily predictors of how humans would react to the same test circumstances. Nor is one's personal experience necessarily a predictor of outcomes for other persons. One must, therefore, develop the habit of weighing the evidence when some new miracle diet or nutritional cure is proclaimed. If there is one rule-of-thumb that experience has proven usually to be true, it is that *extremes—either excesses or deficits—usually prove harmful in the long run.*

To evaluate your own nutritional well-being, each of the above factors will need to be considered. In the next chapter, we will take a look at your daily nutritional requirements and how you meet them. Topics such as vegetarianism, health foods, and diet plans will also be discussed. Later on we tackle the problem of overweight, then we will discuss special problems such as atherosclerosis, diabetes, acne, and even food poisoning—conditions in which diet may play an important role. At the end we give recipes for evening meals that can be converted to lunchbox ideas with a difference. The Appendix contains a detailed discussion of specific nutrient requirements.

The Commonsense Guide to Good Eating

After covering this material, you will have a basis for comparing your present eating habits with your body's actual requirements. If there is a difference between the two, you will then be in a position to remedy the situation if you need or choose to do so.

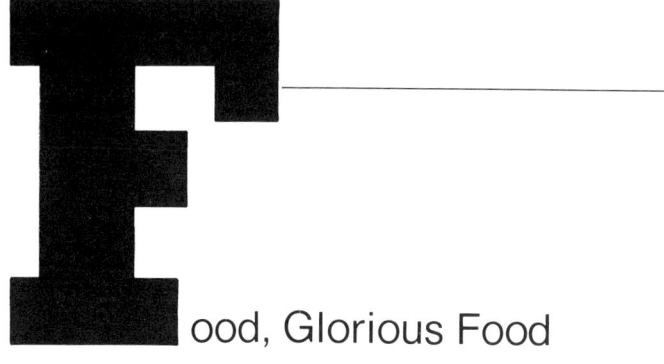ood, Glorious Food

A Discussion of Your Nutrient Requirements

Almost all foods are a mixture of proteins, fats, carbohydrates, vitamins, minerals, water, and indigestible roughage—but in varying amounts. And we have need of all these nutrients, but in fairly well defined proportions. In this chapter we will look at each of these nutrient needs, but first let's see how these recommended allowances are determined.

What Are Recommended Dietary Allowances?

The Recommended Dietary Allowances (RDA)—see Table 1—are the levels of intake of essential nutrients considered, in the judgment of the Food and Nutrition Board of the National Academy of Sciences, on the basis of available scientific knowledge, to be adequate to meet the known nutritional needs of practically all healthy persons for a given age and sex. According to the National Academy of Sciences:[1]

> RDA are presented as daily allowances in order to simplify calculations of nutritional needs. Nevertheless, the various protective mechanisms of the body are such that, if the recommended dietary allowance for a nutrient is not met on a particular day, a surplus consumed shortly thereafter will compensate for the inadequacy. It would seem entirely acceptable, in estimating dietary adequacy, to average intakes of nutrients over a 5-8 day period. However, if nutrient intake is insufficient to meet requirements for a prolonged period, the ability to respond to stress is lessened, and depletion and deterioration eventually occur—despite the effectiveness of the various mechanisms that prolong survival.

The Commonsense Guide to Good Eating

TABLE 1
RECOMMENDED DIETARY ALLOWANCES (RDA)[1,2]

	Age (years)	Weight (kg)	Weight (lbs)	Height (cm)	Height (in)	Energy (kcal)	Protein (gm)	Vitamin A Activity (RE)[3]	Vitamin A Activity (IU)[4]	Vitamin D (IU)	Vitamin E Activity (IU)	Ascorbic Acid (mg)
Infants	0.0-0.5	6	14	60	24	kg x 117	kg x 2.2	420	1,400	400	4	35
	0.5-1.0	9	20	71	28	kg x 108	kg x 2.0	400	2,000	400	5	35
Children	1-3	13	28	86	34	1300	23	400	2,000	400	7	40
	4-6	20	44	110	44	1800	30	500	2,500	400	9	40
	7-10	30	66	135	54	2400	36	700	3,300	400	10	40
Males	11-14	44	97	158	63	2800	44	1,000	5,000	400	12	45
	15-18	61	134	172	69	3000	54	1,000	5,000	400	15	45
	19-22	67	147	172	69	3000	54	1,000	5,000	400	15	45
	23-50	70	154	172	69	2700	56	1,000	5,000		15	45
	51+	70	154	172	69	2400	56	1,000	5,000		15	45
Females	11-14	44	97	155	62	2400	44	800	4,000	400	12	45
	15-18	54	119	162	65	2100	48	800	4,000	400	12	45
	19-22	58	128	162	65	2100	46	800	4,000	400	12	45
	23-50	58	128	162	65	2000	46	800	4,000		12	45
	51+	58	128	162	65	1800	46	800	4,000		12	45
Pregnant						+300	+30	1,000	5,000	400	15	60
Lactating						+500	+20	1,200	6,000	400	15	80

	Folacin[5] (μg)	Niacin (mg)	Riboflavin (mg)	Thiamin (mg)	Vitamin B_6 (mg)	Vitamin B_{12} (μg)	Calcium (mg)	Phosphorus (mg)	Iodine (μg)	Iron (mg)	Magnesium (mg)	Zinc (mg)
Infants	50	5	0.4	0.3	0.3	0.3	360	240	35	10	60	3
	50	8	0.6	0.5	0.4	0.3	540	400	45	15	70	5
Children	100	9	0.8	0.7	0.6	1.0	800	800	60	15	150	10
	200	12	1.1	0.9	0.9	1.5	800	800	80	10	200	10
	300	16	1.2	1.2	1.2	2.0	800	800	110	10	250	10
Males	400	18	1.5	1.4	1.6	3.0	1200	1200	130	18	350	15
	400	20	1.8	1.5	2.0	3.0	1200	1200	150	18	400	15
	400	20	1.8	1.5	2.0	3.0	800	800	140	10	350	15
	400	18	1.6	1.4	2.0	3.0	800	800	130	10	350	15
	400	16	1.5	1.2	2.0	3.0	800	800	110	10	350	15
Females	400	16	1.3	1.2	1.6	3.0	1200	1200	115	18	300	15
	400	14	1.4	1.1	2.0	3.0	1200	1200	115	18	300	15
	400	14	1.4	1.1	2.0	3.0	800	800	100	18	300	15
	400	13	1.2	1.0	2.0	3.0	800	800	100	18	300	15
	400	12	1.1	1.0	2.0	3.0	800	800	80	10	300	15
Pregnant	800	+2	+0.3	+0.3	2.5	4.0	1200	1200	125	18+[6]	450	20
Lactating	600	+4	+0.5	+0.5	2.5	4.0	1200	1200	150	18	450	25

[1] Adapted from Recommended Dietary Allowances, ed 8, publication 2216. Food and Nutrition Board National Research Council 1974. Full report is available from Printing and Publishing Office, National Research Council, 2101 Constitution Avenue, Washington, D.C. 20418 for $2.50.
[2] The allowances are intended to provide for individual variations among most normal persons as they live in the United States under usual environmental stresses. Diets should be based on a variety of common foods in order to provide other nutrients for which human requirements have been less well defined.
[3] Retinol equivalents.
[4] International units
[5] The folacin allowances refer to dietary sources as determined by Lactobacillus casei assay. Pure forms of folacin may be effective in doses less than one-fourth of the RDA.
[6] This increased requirement cannot be met by ordinary diets; therefore, the use of supplemental iron is recommended.

Food, Glorious Food

The RDA for vitamins and minerals are *recommendations* for the amounts of these nutrients that should be consumed daily. RDA should not be confused with *requirements,* however, because there may be differences in the nutritional requirements of specific individuals. It should be stressed, therefore, that even if a person habitually consumes less than the recommended amounts of some nutrients, his or her diet is not necessarily inadequate for those nutrients. However, it is assumed that the further the regular intake drops below the RDA standard for a particular nutrient and the longer the low intake continues, the greater the risk of vitamin or mineral deficiency.

The RDA are not the same as the USRDA (United States Recommended Daily Allowances) — see Table 2 — developed by the Food and Drug Administration for use in the regulation of food labeling for nutritional content. USRDA standards are derived from RDA but, of necessity, are based on very few broad age groups, rather than on the somewhat larger number of age-sex groups for which RDA are established. This means that the RDA are somewhat more tailored requirements than the USRDA. For our purposes, we will refer to the RDA formulated by the National Academy of Sciences.

For some nutrients the recommendation must be based largely on one or two experimental trials on a small number of human subjects. Not only are experiments on human beings costly, they must often be of long duration, and certain types of experiments are not possible for ethical reasons. And even under the best conditions, only a small number of subjects can be studied in a single experiment.

For other nutrients there are so few experiments on human subjects that allowances must be estimated either from information about the requirements of other mammals or from information about the minimum amount of the nutrient known, from food analyses and dietary surveys, to be consumed by apparently healthy people.

Evaluations for some nutrients are expressed in terms of a single part of the nutrient, whereas the recommendation is actually for a composite of the several parts of the nutrient, all of which may differ in efficiency of utilization. Protein intake, for example, is estimated in terms of nitrogen, not specific amino acids; therefore, inefficient utilization of the mixture of amino acids in the protein ingested must be taken into account in developing protein allowances (see Chapter 4 for a complete explanation of this). For some nutrients, absorption may be incomplete; allowance must be made, therefore, for failure of a proportion of the ingested nutrient to gain entrance to the body. Only a small fraction of the iron in foods is absorbed, for example, and this is taken into consideration in developing the recommended allowances.

It is necessary to recognize these problems in order to understand why recommendations for nutrient allowances may differ from country to country and why the allowances for some nutrients exceed the presumed requirement

TABLE 2
U.S. RECOMMENDED DAILY ALLOWANCES (U.S. RDA)
(For use in nutrition labeling of foods, including foods that also are vitamin and mineral supplements)

Nutrient	Adults and Children Over 4 Years	Infants and Children Under 4 Years
Protein	65 gm[1]	28 gm[1]
Vitamin A	5,000 IU	2,500 IU
Vitamic C	60 mg	40 mg
Thiamine	1.5 mg	0.7 mg
Riboflavin	1.7 mg	0.8 mg
Niacin	20 mg	9.0 mg
Calcium	1.0 gm	0.8 gm
Iron	18 mg	10 mg
Vitamin D	400 IU	400 IU
Vitamin E	30 IU	10 IU
Vitamin B_6	2.0 mg	0.7 mg
Folacin	0.4 mg	0.2 mg
Vitamin B_{12}	6 mcg	3 mcg
Phosphorus	1.0 gm	0.8 gm
Iodine	150 mcg	70 mcg
Magnesium	400 mg	200 mg
Zinc	15 mg	8.0 mg
Copper	2 mg	1.0 mg
Biotin	0.3 mg	0.15 mg
Pantothenic Acid	10 mg	5 mg

[1] *If protein efficiency ratio of protein is equal to or better than that of casein. U.S. RDA is 45 gm for adults and 20 gm for infants.*
Source: U.S. Department of Health, Education and Welfare, Public Health Service, Food and Drug Administration, 5600 Fishers Lane, Rockville, Maryland 20852.

by a much greater proportion than those for other nutrients. On the whole, those who accept responsibility for estimating allowances tend to err on the positive side, for there is little evidence that small surpluses of nutrients are detrimental; on the other hand, deficits—even small ones—may lead to deficiencies over a long period of time.

The allowance for energy is treated differenty from allowances for specific nutrients. Energy allowances are based on estimates of the average needs of our population; they are not recommendations for individual intakes, whereas the RDA for vitamins and minerals are recommendations for the amounts that should be consumed daily.

Your Basic Needs

Energy

The body needs energy for its metabolic processes, to support physical activity, growth, production of milk when nursing, and to maintain body temperature. All of these are, therefore, factors in determining an individual's energy needs.

Energy allowances for infants during the first year of life are set at levels reflecting the general pattern of intake of thriving infants and are expressed in terms of *calories*. An allowance of 117 calories per kilogram (54 calories/pound) of body weight has been established for infants at birth, with the allowance decreasing to 100 cals/kg (45 cals/lb) by the end of the first year.

The energy allowances for children of both sexes continue to decline gradually to about 80 cals/kg (36 cals/lb) through ten years of age. After age ten, except for periods of "growth spurt," energy allowances gradually decline further to 45 cals/kg (20 cals/lb) for adolescent males and 38 cals/kg (17 cals/lb) for adolescent females.

Energy requirements decline progressively after early adulthood because the resting metabolic rate declines and growth and physical activity is usually curtailed. It has been proposed that energy allowances for persons above 50 years of age be reduced to 90 percent of the amount required as young adults.

Physical activity is the main variable in estimating energy needs. And since there are wide variations in the physical activity of infants and children as well as adults, energy allowances must be individually adjusted. In Chapter 6, Weight Evaluation and Regulation, we discuss in detail the determination of caloric allowances.

Protein

Protein supplies the amino acids and nitrogen necessary for growth and tissue maintenance. Cells must constantly be repaired and replaced. For example, red blood cells have a life span of only about 120 days; the lining of the small intestine is renewed every one or two days! Therefore, it is obvious that a supply of protein must be maintained. Additionally, extreme environmental or physiological stress increases protein loss and there is evidence that less severe stress may do so as well.

Infections, fevers, and surgical trauma can result in substantial protein loss and greatly increased energy expenditure. Severe infections and surgery should be treated as special conditions that require dietary treatment. During convalescence from an illness that has led to protein depletion, requirements for both protein and energy are elevated for the repletion of wasted tissues, just as they are during periods of rapid growth.

No added allowance is made in the National Academy of Sciences' Recommended Dietary Allowances for the usual stresses encountered in daily living; it is assumed that the subjects of the experiments forming the basis for the requirement estimates are usually exposed to the same stresses as the population generally. Nevertheless, the fact that they point out that the possibility that environmental factors, such as nondisabling infections and the cumulative minor stresses of life in a competitive society, may increase nutritional needs deserves consideration.

It is important to realize that foods differ in quality, quantity, and digestibility. Some protein foods, for example, do not contain all of the necessary amino acids required for growth, maintenance, and repair. In general, animal proteins are more complete sources of amino acids than vegetable proteins. Excessive amounts of animal proteins should not be added to your diet, however. The saturated fatty acid content of meats, when taken over prolonged periods, may be associated with certain types of heart disease. This is discussed later in this chapter and also in the chapter, Atherosclerosis — Prevention Begins at an Early Age.

Eggs, milk, cheese, fish, meat, and poultry all rate very high in biologic value; that is, the completeness of their amino acid patterns plus their digestibility. Of distinctly lower value are the plant proteins such as those of wheat, corn, rice, beans, and nuts. Such incomplete proteins must be supplemented with other foods supplying the missing amino acids in order to provide quality protein. This will be discussed thoroughly in Chapter 4, Vegetarianism — Fad or "a Different Way"?

As you can thus imagine, it is difficult to set "standards" of protein requirements, not only because of the differences in biologic value of the various food proteins, but also because of the differences in human biologic factors such as genetic makeup, endocrine activity, and metabolic efficiency. Then, too, the amounts needed for growth are much greater than those needed for maintenance. Children, for example, need less total protein than adults, but more in proportion to body weight. Infants need approximately 2.2 grams of protein per kilogram (per 2.2 pounds) of body weight, whereas growing adolescents require approximately 1 gram per kilogram of body weight. Adults require 0.8 grams per kilogram for maintenance.

In general, it is safe to say that your supply of quality protein will be ensured if your daily diet includes three average servings of meat, milk, fish, poultry, eggs, or other protein-rich foods such as peas, beans, peanuts, or cheese. This will add up to from 30 to 50 grams of protein. Another 15 to

20 grams of protein will probably be supplied by the grain products and other vegetables needed to round out your caloric requirements. You will not receive any health or energy "bonus" for exceeding this amount.

Fats

Fat is used for energy reserves, internal organ padding, and heat production. It is also required for the absorption of vitamins A, D, E, and K—the "fat-soluble" vitamins.

Fats provide from forty to forty-five percent of the calories in most American diets; this is greatly in excess of physiologic requirements and moderately in excess of the amount felt to be advisable for those leading physically inactive lives. Actually, a well-balanced diet need contain no more than fifteen percent fat. Of more importance than the actual amount of fat consumed, is the type of fat consumed, so let's take a look at the different kinds of fats.

Dietary fats can be divided into two major groups pending on the number of chemical bonds in their carbon chains and their ability to hold hydrogen. If the fat has all single bonds and is, thus, holding all the hydrogen that it can, the fat is said to be *saturated*. If the fat has one or more double bonds and is capable of taking on more hydrogen than it already holds, it is said to be *unsaturated*. As you might expect, unsaturated fats can be subdivided depending on how many double bonds they have: *monounsaturated* fats have only one double bond, and *polyunsaturated* fats have more than one double bond. The following diagram illustrates such bonding.

Now, what's the importance of all this? Fats or foods consisting of primarily saturated fatty acids, when taken in excess over prolonged periods, may raise the blood's cholesterol level. High cholesterol levels are associated with the degenerative blood vessel process known as atherosclerosis and with heart disease. Fats or foods consisting primarily of unsaturated fatty acids do not raise cholesterol levels, and the polyunsaturates actually may tend to help the body get rid of newly formed cholesterol. More information about cholesterol is given in the chapter, Atherosclerosis—Prevention Begins at an Early Age.

Your chances for good health will be greatly improved if you limit your intake of dietary fats to thirty to thirty-five percent of your total calories, no more than ten percent coming from saturated fats. Of the remaining twenty to twenty-five percent, at least ten percent should be from polyunsaturated fats.

The easiest way to remember which fats are saturated and which are unsaturated is to keep in mind that, in general, saturated fats are solid at room temperature—butter, fats in meat, coconut oil, cocoa butter—whereas unsaturated fats are liquid at room temperature—most vegetable oils.

Vegetable oils are unsaturated (except for coconut and palm oils which are highly saturated) and contain no cholesterol. Not all vegetable oils are

The Commonsense Guide to Good Eating

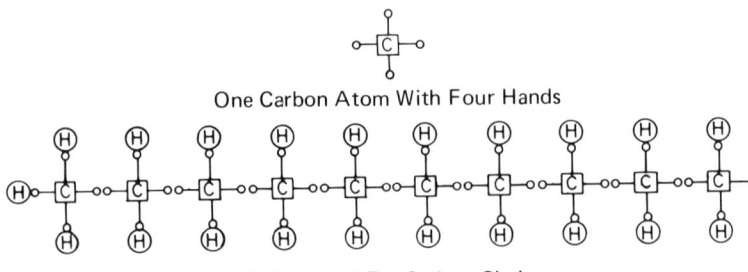

One Carbon Atom With Four Hands

A Saturated Fat Carbon Chain

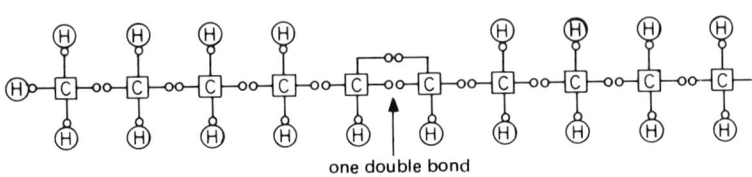

one double bond

A Monounsaturated Fat Carbon Chain

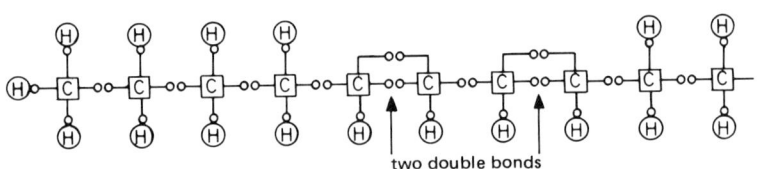

two double bonds

A Polyunsaturated Fat Carbon Chain

polyunsaturated; safflower, soybean, corn, cottonseed, and sesame seed oils are polyunsaturated, whereas olive and peanut oils are monounsaturated.

Beware of the coconut and palm oils lurking in commerical products such as substitute dairy products; cake, cookie, muffin, and pancake mixes; and potato and corn chips. These ingredients are usually labeled simply as "vegetable oil." Do not buy packages that don't specify which oil they contain if you are trying to control your intake.

What about margarine? Vegetable oils can be turned into solids by the addition of hydrogen atoms. The "hydrogenation" changes the unsaturated oils into saturated or partially saturated products. Unless the product is labeled, you will not know what percentage of the margarine is saturated and how much remains unsaturated. An artificially saturated product has absolutely no advantages over a naturally saturated product. A saturated fat is a saturated fat, regardless of how it got that way.

Another term that you may run across is *polyunsaturated-saturated (P/S) ratio*. This is a measure used to gauge the proper intake of fats and is arrived at by dividing the weight of the polyunsaturated fat (P) in your diet or food by the weight of the saturated fat (S). The higher the ratio, the better off you are. The quotient, at the very least, should be "one"; that would mean one part unsaturated fat to one part saturated fat. For example, the P/S value of safflower oil is 9.0, whereas it is 0.6 for olive oil.

One of the problems you will run into in trying to limit your intake of fats is that there are so many "invisible" sources. Nuts, for example, are approximately sixty percent fat. Peanut butter is fifty percent fat; cheese is thirty to thirty-five percent fat; hot dogs and luncheon meats are twenty-five to thirty percent fat; cakes, pies, and ice cream average twelve to thirteen percent fat; and fish is from six to eight percent fat. And don't be fooled by the label "all-beef hotdogs." That doesn't mean that they are one-hundred percent meat; it only means that what meat there is in them is beef and not some other meat.

It is interesting that the presence of fat in food delays the emptying of the stomach. This may contribute to the continued feeling of fullness and lack of hunger after eating a meal rich in fat. Exactly how much fat is required for this isn't apparent, but most low-calorie diets include at least some fat for this reason. Also, as mentioned previously, some fat is necessary for the absorption of the "fat-soluble" vitamins.

Carbohydrates

Carbohydrates provide most of the energy in almost all human diets. Carbohydrates also play an interesting role in assisting the body to utilize proteins in the most efficient manner. This is important for two reasons: 1) sources of protein are usually expensive, and 2) though the body can derive carbohydrates from protein, the body's store of protein is dependent solely on what is taken in as protein. Thus, you don't want the proteins sidetracked into activities that can be performed by more readily available and, hence, less expensive foods. This is especially important with today's high meat prices and the large number of families with marginal incomes.

Indiscriminate addition of carbohydrates to the diet is to be avoided, however. There is good evidence to suggest that the increasing use of sugar — one type of carbohydrate — by Americans has contributed to the growing incidence of degenerative blood vessel disease, especially when the sugar is combined with excessive amounts of animal fats. Unfortunately, people who eat fat-rich diets usually also eat excessive amounts of sugar.

The principal carbohydrates in foods are sugars, starches, and cellulose. The sugars include the monosaccharides and disaccharides in refined sugars, jams, jellies, syrups, honey, fruits, and milk. The starches are the polysaccharides of cereals, flour, potatoes, and other vegetables. The more complex carbohydrates, such as cellulose, are largely indigestible but are important in providing bulk in the diet and aiding bowel elimination.

Vitamins and minerals

The National Academy of Sciences lists a number of vitamins and minerals which may eventually prove essential for the maintenance of good health. However, present knowledge about human needs limits setting daily allowances to ten vitamins and six minerals. The amounts recommended are designed to afford a margin of safety above average physiological requirements to cover variation among individuals in the population. It must be remembered, however, that infections, even mild ones, increase losses of many valuable nutrients and this at a time when poor appetite may lead to an even greater depletion of body stores. In addition, acute or chronic infections involving the gastrointestinal tract may impair the absorption of nutrients.

The exact amounts of vitamins and minerals required depend on your state of health, your body size, and whether you are rapidly growing, menstruating, pregnant, or nursing a baby. Hence, requirements are different for males and females of the same age. In reviewing the Recommended Daily Dietary Allowances, you will notice that no distinction is made between the sexes up to age ten, since weight ranges are not very different for males and females up to this age, and factors such as menstruation and pregnancy usually have not yet entered the picture.

Some vitamins and minerals known to be required by the body are either synthesized by the body and/or are required in such minute amounts that there seems to be no likelihood of a deficiency.

In addition to the natural occurrence of certain vitamins and minerals in various foods, some foods are artificially *enriched* or *fortified*. Enriched and fortified both refer to the addition of specific nutrients to foods, but there is a difference. *Enrichment* usually refers to the addition of one or more nutrients to a food to bring it back to the level it was before the nutrients were lost in processing! *Enriched* is a very misleading word it seems.

The amounts and variety of nutrients added to *fortified* products are usually in excess of those normally found in the food because of the importance of providing additional amounts of the nutrients to the diet. Some foods are selected for fortification because they are an appropriate carrier for the specific nutrient. For example, milk is frequently fortified with vitamin D. Vitamin D improves the body's utilization of the calcium and phosphorus found in milk.

We should say a few words about vitamins and minerals before we consider how much of each you need. Vitamins are classified as either fat-soluble

Food, Glorious Food

or water-soluble. There are four fat-soluble vitamins: A, D, E, and K. The nine "B-complex" vitamins and vitamin C are water-soluble.

Fat-soluble vitamins are found in fatty animal products such as egg yolk, butter, cream, meat fats, and fish oils, but are also present in vegetable oils. Water-soluble vitamins, other than vitamin B_{12}, are found in varying amounts in all green leafy vegetables, yeast, seed germs and, except for vitamin C, in lean animal meat. Organ meats such as liver and kidneys are especially rich in their vitamin B_{12} content.

Fat-soluble vitamins are less likely to be lost in cooking than water-soluble vitamins because they are more stable in the presence of heat. Water-soluble vitamins, being soluble in water and somewhat sensitive to heat, are lost in large quantities during the cooking process. For example, up to sixty percent of the vitamin C content of green leafy and yellow vegetables can be lost during cooking.

Fat-soluble vitamins are absorbed from the intestine along with fats and, thus, anything that interferes with fat absorption also interferes with utilization of these vitamins. Because these vitamins are not soluble in water, they are not excreted in the urine and, thus, are stored in the body. This is a very important point because it means that too much of these vitamins can accumulate and toxicity — a poisonous state — can develop.

The dangers of excessive vitamin-mineral intake are not widely known, and the advertisements for super-vitamins and vitamin-rich products do nothing to correct this. Probably unintentionally, many food and drug companies give the impression that if a little bit is good, a lot has to be better. Who can blame the child bombarded by this kind of message on the television for scooping up a handful of vitamins made to look like candy or his favorite TV cartoon character? Vitamin poisoning is second only to aspirin poisoning in young children!

Excesses of the water-soluble vitamins are not usually stored in the body but are excreted in the urine; hence, toxicity does not usually occur. Since there is little or no storage of most of these vitamins, care must be taken to replace them daily, especially during periods of illness when losses are accentuated. It is of concern that sugar and pure fats, which supply a large percentage of the energy intake of the average American's diet, provide *no* water-soluble vitamins.

One of the main things to keep in mind about vitamins is that even though several vitamins may be involved in a seemingly identical function, lack of any one of the vitamins involved will retard the function. For example, vitamins A, B^1, B^6, C, and D are all involved in stimulating growth. When any one of these vitamins is supplied in inadequate amounts, growth will be stunted, even though the food contains plenty of the other vitamins needed for growth.

Minerals and trace elements differ from each other in respect to the amount required by the body. For example, the macrominerals calcium, phosphorus, and magnesium are required in amounts greatly in excess of the trace elements iron, iodine, and zinc.

Many vitamins and minerals are interrelated and dependent upon one another. Phosphorus is a good example of this phenomenon. Not only must the intake of phosphorus and calcium be reasonably balanced for each to maintain its proper function, but many of the B vitamins are effective only when combined with phosphorus.

We're not sure that you really need—let alone want—to know what each vitamin and mineral does. However, you will find in the Appendix a concise discussion of each vitamin, mineral, and trace element should you be interested.

The recent U.S. Health and Nutrition Survey showed that segments of our population are at risk for various nutrient deficiencies. There are, however, many who question the findings and their interpretation. Some people feel that the sample population was too small to justify some of the conclusions drawn. The report published thus far is only a preliminary one and the National Center for Health Statistics plans to expand the study to include other states and populations. When the final report is available, it is hoped that more meaningful conclusions can be drawn concerning the nutritional well-being of our citizens.

Water

Though water has no caloric value, it is a most important nutrient. Water stands next to air in importance to life. You can get along for days, even weeks, without food but you will survive only a few days without water.

Water is necessary for all the processes of digestion. Additionally, nutrients are dissolved in water so that they may pass through the intestinal wall and into the blood stream for use throughout the body. Water carries waste out of the body, and water also helps to regulate body temperature.

The body's most obvious source of water is the water that a person drinks, but there are many other sources as well. Soup is a water source, as are many fruits and vegetables. Even meat can be up to eighty percent water.

The multitude of factors determining water loss preclude setting a minimal water requirement. Under normal circumstances, however, a reasonable minimum adult amount would be about one quart per day. Thirst is a pretty good indicator of need for the healthy adult, but is not a reliable sign during illness or once dehydration is established, especially in infants and young children.

Special attention must be given to the water needs of the following individuals: infants on high-protein formulas and of others consuming high protein diets; those with fever, vomiting, or diarrhea; individuals taking diuretics; athletes and persons in hot and humid environments; and unconscious patients.

Roughage

The indigestible residues of fruits, vegetables, and grains are often referred to as roughage, fiber, bulk, or cellulose. These residues contribute little or nothing of nutritional value, but are exceedingly necessary for the proper functioning of the lower intestinal tract and for the formation of feces and the prevention of constipation.

It has also been observed that the incidence of cancer of the colon is lower in populations where the diet is based on coarse cereals with a high fiber content. With such diets, the feces pass through the colon rapidly. With diets low in roughage, the colonic contents tend to stagnate and this may change the bacterial flora. It is theorized that in this way, carcinogens may be produced by bacteria within the lumen of the bowel.

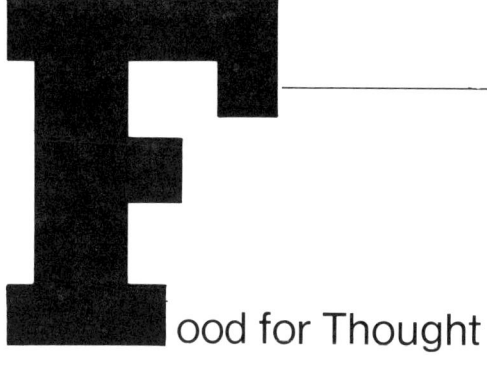ood for Thought

Five Goals, Plus Information About Eating Habits

Nutritional problems are essentially educational, economic, and behavioral problems. We have the world's greatest food production system, but often we don't possess enough knowledge to make wise, nutritionally sound choices. Food selection should be based on meeting at least five goals: to satisfy your nutrient and health requirements; to achieve a caloric value in accordance with your weight plan; to purchase foods at a price compatible with your budget; to satisfy your taste and visual senses; and to stop your hunger pangs. In this chapter we will look at each one of these goals, but first let's consider some of the things that influence our eating behavior.

Eating Habits

Food habits and attitudes are fashioned very early in life; many are good and are intentionally fostered by parents, but some are bad and are unintentionally determined. For example, consider the effect of withholding dessert as a form of punishment for bad behavior or using it as a reward for "cleaning your plate." Either way, dessert is likely to assume undue importance and may be the beginning of a "sweet tooth." Likewise, using a bottle or other food as a pacifier to distract a fussy child may well set the stage for the development of a pattern of eating when bored or under stress, not to mention the deleterious effects on the baby's first teeth from the constant half-filled bottle of milk in the baby's mouth—"nursing bottle syndrome."

Food preferences also get established rather early in life. One woman served her children steak every night because "that's all they like." When the children were asked why they wouldn't eat hamburger, they replied that it was because it was never served to them! Of course, there's the other side of the coin: being made to eat spinach because "it's good for you" has resulted in a lot of adult spinach haters.

It's also important to remember that people's tastes change. You may genuinely hate broccoli today, but five years from now you may find that it's not so bad—especially when served with hollandaise sauce rather than plain. Likewise, you may grow tired of an old favorite. There's nothing wrong with either situation, but tasting every now and then a once disliked or tired-of food or a dish you've never tried can keep your menu from becoming a bore.

Ethnic influences and economic considerations also play a tremendous role in determining the foods served and eaten. Spaghetti and macaroni are a delicious staple found in many homes. The presence of this foodstuff may relate to the family's dietary preference or it might be used as a menu stretcher because it is relatively inexpensive. When discussing "good eating habits," it would be foolish to ignore food preference and cost.

Pediatricians often refer to the grandmothers of America as the single most powerful organization affecting the nutritional well-being of children. Since our educational system doesn't prepare young men and women for the care and feeding of infants, new parents must rely heavily on the advice of their own parents. Unfortunately, the myth that "a fat baby is a healthy baby" is still with us, as is the "join the clean plate club" slogan. Years ago, it used to be "eat everything on your plate—the children in Europe are starving."

Physicians must shoulder their share of the blame, too: "Feed the baby four ounces of milk *every* four hours"; "Give the child small amounts so he will learn to *clean* his plate." Better communication between physicians and parents is clearly called for. Instructions meant as guidelines are only too often carried out "to the letter." How many times have you seen a young parent awaken an infant so that it will finish its bottle? Too often, unfortunately.

Breast-feeding would be a boon to future generations if for no other reason than the mother wouldn't be able to see how many ounces of milk the baby had taken and, thus, wouldn't be tempted to feed the baby more than he needed to feel satisfied!

Three meals a day?

Not necessarily, and not even ideally. There is nothing inherently right about eating three times a day, or wrong about multiple snacks rather than three basic meals. Nutritional deficiencies can occur regardless of the number or size of the meals. Actually, most nutritional difficulties arise when the individual eats fewer than three times a day—which brings us to the subject of breakfast, the meal most often omitted.

It is the feeling of many lay and professional nutrition people that breakfast is the most important meal of the day. Their reasoning is that the prolonged

Food for Thought

period of fasting while sleeping subjects the body to low blood sugar levels, and unless adequate nourishment is taken the blood sugar level continues to fall, resulting in a decrease in efficiency and attention span in school or at work during the late morning hours. Others say that breakfast isn't necessary, that it's a matter of habit, and that if you give yourself a few days to adjust to not eating breakfast that you'll feel just fine.

Who's right? A person's eating habits are the product of so many variables—cultural, economic, food preferences and attitudes, family or peer patterns, time and food available, etc.—that it is probably more reasonable to decide what best fits your life-style and makes you feel best than to try and establish a norm by which all should be measured.

To help you decide whether breakfast is or is not for you, here are some of the more often quoted arguments for both sides. In the end, however, you should choose the eating pattern that causes the least family friction—in some families group eating is more important than in others—and yet is compatible with your preferences and time schedule.

What are the "pros" of eating breakfast? If you're on a reducing diet and are, understandably, constantly thinking about food, you may find that the sacrifice of skipping breakfast or lunch just succeeds in making you ravenous at the next meal. What's the result? You guessed it, overeating! If you're trying to gain weight, you probably need this meal to help you take in all the necessary calories.

One authority maintains that if you're not hungry in the morning it's because you ate too much the night before and that calories taken in prior to a dormant or inactive period such as sleep will cause fat to accumulate more readily than the same number of calories taken in but followed by activity. The advice there might be interpreted as eat a large breakfast and a very light dinner.

What about the "cons" of eating breakfast? Probably the worst thing about breakfast is the kind of foods people choose to eat. To quote Dr. Laurence E. Lamb, from his book *What You Need to Know About Food and Cooking for Health,* "Add to the cholesterol in two eggs the fat in bacon and the butter on the toast, and you will find you are starting the day with far too much fat of any kind, saturated fat in particular, and insulting the principle of health by exceeding the entire daily allowance for cholesterol. No wonder Americans have one of the highest incidences of fatty deposits in their arteries of any people on the earth."[1]

Those who favor the breakfast route say that the meal should contain one-fourth of your daily protein allowance. Those opposed to breakfast say if you're going to eat it, learn to eat more healthful foods—fish, for example. An obvious compromise is a light, low-calorie, low-fat breakfast of juice and cereal with skim milk and fruit when available.

The Commonsense Guide to Good Eating

Nutritional do's and don'ts

The following is a concise listing of do's and don'ts that will help you establish and maintain good eating habits.

DO	DON'T
Eat three servings of protein-rich foods a day. Protein is required for growth and body maintenance. No other nutrient can act as a substitute.	Omit carbohydrates from your diet. They aid in the efficient use of proteins. This is especially important when the price of protein foods minimizes your protein intake. Carbohydrates also protect you from ketosis, an abnormal situation that is very dangerous for some.
Limit your intake of fats to 30% of your total daily calories. A good balance would be: 10% saturated, 10% monounsaturated, and 10% polyunsaturated. Excessive amounts of saturated fats may be dangerous to your long-term health.	Take more than the recommended daily allowances of vitamins and minerals. Some are poisonous in large amounts.
See that your daily vitamin and mineral intake is adequate. Prolonged deficiencies can strip your body of its natural defenses against disease, especially during periods of growth such as in adolescence and pregnancy.	Become a heavy salt eater. An increased incidence of high blood pressure has been noted in heavy salt users.
Try to reach and maintain your ideal weight. You'll look better, feel better, and be healthier.	Take in more than 300 mg of cholesterol a day. High blood serum cholesterol levels are associated with an increased incidence of heart and vascular disease. The American Heart Association suggests that you eat no more than three egg yolks — a rich source of cholesterol — a week.
Know that three meals a day is not necessarily better than snacking. It's the overall quality and quantity of food eaten that's important — not the time when you eat it.	Exceed your proper daily caloric allowance. Overweight people have more health problems than others.

In general, it is felt that if your daily diet includes as a minimum the following foods, your nutrient needs will be adequately protected:
- *8 ounces of vitamin D-fortified milk:* this is to protect your calcium, phosphorus, magnesium, vitamins A, D, B_{12} and riboflavin reserves, as well as to provide protein.
- *2 servings of meat, fish, poultry, eggs, or cheese:* these provide protein, iron, and B vitamins.
- *1 citrus fruit:* vitally needed to protect your vitamin C requirements.
- *1 serving of a dark green or deep yellow vegetable at least every other day:* this supplies vitamin A and some iron.

- *1 serving of bread or cereal:* this provides carbohydrates, vitamin B-complex, and iron.

These foods can, of course, be put together in a variety of ways. Cereal with fruit and milk for breakfast, a cheeseburger and a milkshake for lunch, and a green pepper stuffed with tuna salad for dinner is a pretty nutritious feast!

When time, money, illness, etc., prevent you from getting your protein, vitamins, and minerals through a variety of foods, you may want to consider a protein and vitamin-mineral supplement.

Hints for when you dine out

Eating out is often a problem for the diet-minded person. For example, what do you choose when you're trying to restrict your caloric intake or when you're trying to reduce the amount of saturated fat in your diet?

For one thing, try to avoid fried foods, foods covered with batter or sauces, or foods that are a mixture of unidentifiable things, such as a meat loaf or croquettes. If you have a choice, pick fish, chicken, turkey, veal, or very lean beef; refuse or discard any crust, skin, or sauce that comes with it. Any soup or vegetable that starts with *cream of* or *creamed* should be avoided, as should vegetables cooked or served with fats such as fat-back or butter.

What do you have for dessert? Consider fresh fruit, angel food cake, jello, or sherbert. Puddings, chocolate desserts, eclairs, and doughnuts are poor choices.

How to Be Calorie Wise, Not Pound Foolish

As noted earlier, nearly all foods are a mixture of proteins, fats, carbohydrates, minerals, vitamins, water, and indigestible roughage. Because of this varying composition of foods, different foods have different caloric values. For example, look at some of the differences in the foods in Table 3.

Compare the composition of the applesauce with that of the canned apricots. Notice how much alike they are and how close they are in calories? Other than their water content, most of their weight is from carbohydrates. *Every gram of carbohydrate contains about four calories.* Actually, the caloric value of carbohydrates varies from 3.6 calories per gram in fruits to 4.12 in certain cereals.

Now, compare the applesauce and the apriots with yet another fruit, the avocado. The avocado has about the same amount of water, but much less of its weight comes from carbohydrates. But look at its fat content and calorie count! Fat, obviously, is higher caloried than carbohydrates; in fact, it has more than twice the calories. *Every gram of fat contains about nine calories.* Again, there is a range of actual values—from 8.37 for fruits and vegetables up to 9.02 for meat, fish, and eggs.

TABLE 3
COMPARISON OF FOUR FOODS

Food 100 grams (3.5 oz) of each	Amount of Weight (in grams)					
	Proteins	Fats	Carbohydrates	Water	Other	Calories
Applesauce	0.2	0.1	23.8	75.7	0.2	91
Apricots, canned	0.6	0.1	22.0	76.9	1.3	86
Avocados	2.2	17.0	6.0	73.6	1.2	171
Flounder	16.7	0.8	-	81.3	1.2	79

Look at the flounder. Other than its water content, most of its weight comes from proteins. Notice how similar the caloric value of the flounder is to that of the applesauce and the apricots? Like carbohydrates, *every gram of protein contains approximately four calories.* Protein varies in caloric value, too—from 3.11 in vegetables to 4.36 in eggs.

A food's total caloric value depends on the number of calories from protein, the number of calories from fats, and the number of calories from carbohydrates. Let's look at another example—a glass of whole milk versus a glass of low-fat or skim milk—Table 4.

You will notice that the number of calories coming from proteins, for example, is exactly the same for both the whole milk and the low-fat milk, yet the total caloric value of the two milks is dramatically different. The difference is directly attributable to the amount of fat. Remember, fat contains about twice the amount of calories as does either protein or carbohydrate. Reducing the amount of fat in the milk can cut the number of total calories almost in half, without reducing the protein value.

As you can see, you can greatly affect your caloric intake by your choice of foods. Potato chips obviously have a lot more calories than carrot sticks, but what about something less obvious? Consider the different cuts of beef, for example.

Cut of Beef	Fat Content	Calories per Ounce
Flank steak	almost none	41
T-bone steak	38%	113
Ground round, trimmed of fat	5%	38
Ground chuck, trimmed of fat	7%	45
Regular ground beef	25-30%	86-100

And don't let the higher cost-per-pound for lean meats keep you from considering them. Remember, you get more servings from lean meat because there's no fat to melt away and go to waste. You're also doing your health a favor by restricting your intake of saturated fat.

TABLE 4
COMPOSITION OF MILK [1]

	Whole Milk[2]	Low-fat Milk[2]
Proteins		
grams	7.0	7.0
calories	29.89	29.89
Fats		
grams	7.8	0.2
calories	68.56	1.76
Carbohydrates		
grams	9.8	10.2
calories	37.93	39.47
Water		
grams	174	181
calories	-	-
Other		
grams	1.4	1.6
calories	-	-
Total		
grams	200	200
calories	136.38	71.12

[1] These values were arrived at by multiplying the number of grams of protein, fat, and carbohydrate by their specific caloric value in milk (4.27, 8.79, 3.87 respectively). It would have come within one calorie of the correct total calories had we used the slightly less accurate caloric values of 4 for proteins and carbohydrates and 9 for fats. For most practical purposes, and certainly for ease in remembering, 4 cals/gm protein, 4 cals/gm carbohydrate, and 9 cals/gm fat is accurate enough.
[2] 200 grams (7 ounces) of each.

Vegetables can also be very deceiving in their caloric content. Compare one cup of each of the following:

Vegetable	Calories
Turnip greens	30
Asparagus	36
Beets	50
Baby lima beans	180

Fish? You can save 61 calories per half-cup simply by buying your tuna canned in water rather than in oil.

Cereals? One cup of Kellogg's Special K will cost you only half the calories of Sugar Frosted Flakes—70 calories compared with 143 calories. If you like your cereal sweet and yet must be stingy with the calories, use an artificial sweetener at about 3.5 calories for the sweetness of 2 teaspoons instead of regular sugar which would cost you 30 calories.

Don't forget desserts. A chocolate sundae made with one-half cup ice cream, two tablespoons chocolate sauce, and two tablespoons whipped cream would normally add up to about 300 calories. The same sundae made with low-sugar chocolate sauce and low-calorie whipped topping is only about 150 calories—exactly half of the higher-calorie product.

You can save on cola beverages. Twelve ounces of regular cola will cost you 145 calories, but the same amount of an artificially sweetened cola is only two calories. Look at the wine list, too. Three ounces of a sweet wine are 160 calories, whereas the same amount of dry wine is only 85 calories.

And don't overlook the calorie savings possible on bread. Super-thin slices—often called "melba"—contain about 44 calories compared to regular-size slices at 70 calories.

The food exchange system described in a later chapter will help you protect your vitamin, mineral, protein, etc., needs while allowing you to keep your caloric intake within proper bounds. It is difficult, however, to get all the vitamins and minerals you need in diets of less than 1,200 calories daily. Many physicians recommend a multi-vitamin-mineral supplement for low-calorie dieters.

Trying to gain weight? Read the suggestions in Chapter 6.

Tips for Staying Within Your Food Budget

Without question, prices are at an all-time high—but there are some ways to help bring your food budget into line.

Make a menu and a shopping list and then stick to it; and don't go to the store when you're hungry. Impulse buying is responsible for a sizable chunk of many food dollars.

Use leftovers wisely and promptly. All those dabs of leftover meat and vegetables plus the juice drained off canned or freshly cooked vegetables combine to make a delicious soup.

Use magazine and newspaper coupons if they are for items you will really use. Those saved pennies add up.

Nonfat dry milk is cheaper serving-for-serving than whole milk—yet equally nutritious. A glass of whole fluid milk usually costs three times as much as a

Food for Thought

glass of reconstituted nonfat dry milk. Nonfat dry milk is an excellent source of protein. It will also save on calories. If you don't care for its taste for drinking, you can mix it half-and-half with regular milk or use it for cooking.

Save on day-old bread and cakes, and then extend their lives by storage in the refrigerator or freezer. When the bread is too dry for other uses, crush or cut and toast it for bread crumbs or cubes. Incidentally, dried out bread can be freshened by sprinkling it with water, wrapping it in foil, and warming it gently in the oven.

Compare the cost of supermarket brand foods to name-brand products. They are often, but not always, cheaper. Also, check weekly specials advertised in the local newspaper, but don't use up more money in gasoline, running around to different stores, than you save on the food item.

Is there a food cooperative in your area? The donation of a few hours of your time may save you many food dollars. If there is a college or university nearby, check with the Student Activities Office. They may be able to give you a lead in locating a co-op. Students are often active in such endeavors.

Take advantage of seasonal abundances but limit purchases of perishable items to amounts that can be used while they are at their best.

Buy ready-to-serve cereals in the larger boxes rather than in the individual-sized packages. The small multipacks may cost two or three times more per ounce than the same cereal in a larger box. Also, sugar-coated cereals cost more per ounce than many common unsweetened ones.

Cereals you cook yourself—especially the kinds that take longer to cook—are nearly always less expensive than the ready-prepared ones.

A can of solid white meat tuna costs more than the same size can of grated light meat tuna. You may prefer the solid pack for a salad and the grated pack for casseroles and sandwich fillings.

When considering convenience foods, make sure that the time saved is worth the money lost. Another plus of do-it-yourself foods is that you can usually save on calories and saturated fats as well as money.

Check to see if unsliced luncheon meats and cheese are a better buy than presliced and individually wrapped items. They often are.

Plan more meals based on vegetable proteins. There are a number of good books which contain recipes so delicious you'll wonder why you ever thought *vegetables* meant just buttered carrots or string beans. A few especially good books that not only contain great recipes but which will help you adjust your own recipes to improve their protein efficiency include:

- Lappe, F.M. *Diet for a Small Planet.* New York: Ballantine Books, 1975.
- Ewald, E.B. *Recipes for a Small Planet.* New York: Ballantine Books, 1973.
- Ford, M.W., Hillyard, S., and Koock, M.F. *The Deaf Smith Country Cookbook.* New York: Macmillan, 1973.

Beauty Is in the Eye of the Beholder

Food that looks pretty always seems to taste better. Even a cup of coffee is improved by serving it in a nice mug rather than in a paper cup.

Likewise, a bruised tomato may be a good buy, but it's not very attractive. Better it get used to make tomato sauce than served as is.

Taste and visual appeal are especially important when dealing with a picky eater, but if a person just doesn't like the taste of a food, no amount of dressing will make it appealing. You'd be better off to spend your money on food that is really enjoyed and won't be wasted.

Stopping the Hunger Pangs

Many weight regulation diets fail because they just don't seem to stop the hunger pangs. It's hard to think about anything but food when your stomach is growling! The food exchange system in Chapter 7 will help you identify satisfying but low-calorie foods. Also, the diet plans accompanying the food exchange lists allow for mid-afternoon and late-evening snacks*.

The diet plans and food exchange lists will also prove useful to those trying to gain weight, as well as to those who want to otherwise improve their nutrient intake.

---

*Some studies suggest that food eaten late in the day may turn to fat, whereas food eaten earlier in the day is efficiently utilized. This has importance for both those trying to lose and trying to gain weight.

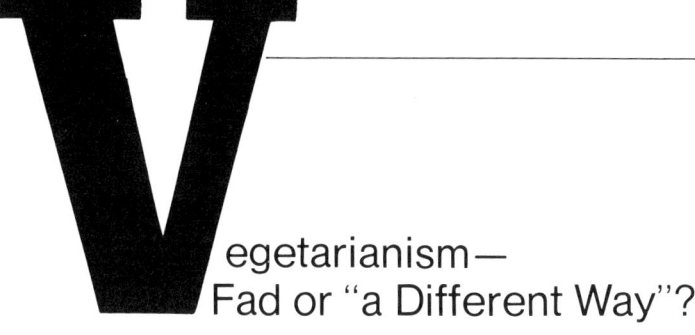
Vegetarianism— Fad or "a Different Way"?

The Problems and the Benefits

There are many degrees of vegetarianism, ranging from lacto-ovo-vegetarians who use eggs and dairy products such as milk, cheese, and butter but who exclude meat from their diet to mono-vegetarians who eat only one food, such as brown rice. There are also many reasons for these dietary preferences.

Many vegetarians hold that life in all forms is sacred, and that all creatures have the right to live out their normal life span. Others maintain that animal meats are not healthy, that they're being injected with too many hormones and antibiotics. Still others say that it takes more land to raise livestock and their feed than it does to raise grain for humans; hence, a wasteful use of our limited space—an important consideration in a world rapidly becoming overpopulated. Then, too, some groups adhere to a vegetable diet because of the high cost of meat or as part of their religious or spiritual life.

Science can add yet another reason: many studies have reported that vegetarians usually have lower serum cholesterol and triglyceride levels than nonvegetarians, and at least one study showed that a group of male California Seventh-day Adventists (who are lacto-ovo-vegetarians) suffered their first heart attack a full decade later than most Americans, and their incidence of heart disease was only sixty percent of that of the average California male population. For more information about the relationship of diet to heart disease, you may want to refer to the chapter, Atherosclerosis—Prevention Begins at an Early Age.

Vegetarianism has long been popular in Eastern countries where there is a belief in reincarnation, and where cattle are precious and refrigerators are scarce. The cow's sacredness in India has not always been based on compassion and religious beliefs! In the United States, a large number of our young people are avoiding meat for a variety of reasons and are, or probably will be, rearing their children in like fashion. Thus a vegetarian way of life may be followed because of commitment, health, necessity, or a combination of these factors.

By and large, vegetarians are healthy people, suffering from nutritional deficiencies no more—and in some instances, less—than others. If, however, dairy products are avoided in addition to meat, great care is needed to avoid deficiencies in vitamin B_{12}, riboflavin, iron, zinc, and calcium. Vitamin D could also be a problem for children not adequately exposed to sunlight. The biggest problem, however, is to obtain all the necessary amino acids, especially during growth periods.

Special Concerns

Amino acids

Protein supplies the amino acids necessary for growth and tissue maintenance. The body requires a number of different amino acids and, within limits, can actually convert one amino acid into another. There are, however, several amino acids which the body cannot make itself and must be obtained from the diet. These are called the *essential amino acids.*

There are eight essential amino acids required by adults; children require a ninth during growth. Furthermore, since the body has no mechanism for the storage of individual amino acids, all of the essential amino acids must be present at the same meal or within a very brief time interval for any one of them to do its proper job.

The quality of a particular food as a protein source is not only related to its digestibility and absorption but also to whether or not it contains all the essential amino acids. At the top of the list of quality protein foods is egg; next comes milk. Both egg and milk proteins can furnish all the amino acids essential for normal growth and healthy life processes provided they are eaten in sufficient amounts.

Fish, meat, and poultry are also quality protein sources. Of distinctly lower quality are the plant proteins such as those in wheat, corn, rice, beans, and nuts. These plant proteins may contain all the necessary amino acids, but in each one of them one or more of the essential amino acids is present in such inadequate amounts that the entire protein value is diminished. The deficient amino acid is sometimes referred to as the "limiting" amino acid— that is, it limits your body's utilization of the protein. There is a way around this problem, however.

If a protein food is missing or low in one or more of the essential amino acids, the deficiency can be made up by eating—at or near the same meal, don't forget—another food which contains the missing elements. This process is called "mutual supplementation" or "protein complementarity." Mutual supplementation of proteins has been practiced instinctively for ages, though its nutritional importance has been recognized only in this century. Examples of mutual supplementation include: macaroni and cheese, bread and milk, beans and rice, corn and beans, breakfast cereal with milk, peanut butter and bread.

Supplementation of cereal proteins with synthetic amino acids offers hope for coping with worldwide food problems. More research into the area of amino acid nutrition will be needed, however, before synthetic supplementation can become a widely approved and accepted procedure.

In general, legumes and leafy vegetables (for example, peas, beans, lentils, peanuts, greens) quite adequately supplement grains: wheat, oat, corn, rye, barley, rice. But if your diet merely avoids animal flesh but does include dairy products, all the essential amino acids will most probably be supplied without your ever having to worry about it. If, however, dairy products are also avoided, care must be taken to avoid serious nutritional problems. A general rule of thumb is that if seventy percent of the protein in the diet comes from wheat protein and thirty percent comes from milk, yeast, nuts, soybeans, and other legumes, there will be excellent supplementary action. Of interest to those who avoid dairy products is the fact that a mixture of soy and sesame proteins has a high nutritive value, comparable to milk proteins.

Milk normally supplies 75 percent of the calcium, 43 percent of the riboflavin, 22 percent of the protein, and practically 100 percent of the vitamin B_{12} in the diet. One way for the pure vegetarian to obtain an adequate intake of these nutrients is to use sufficient quantities of fortified soybean milk. For an adult, this would mean about two glasses a day. The label should be checked to make sure the soybean milk is fortified. Otherwise, a vitamin supplement is probably called for.

Vitamin B_{12}

When all animal products—meat, eggs, milk, cheese, etc.—are eliminated from the diet, the diet will not provide any vitamin B_{12} since this vitamin is found in only the most minute quantities in some plants. This is of critical concern because a vitamin B_{12} deficiency can give rise to pernicious anemia—among other things—which, if not treated, can lead to serious illness and death. Vitamin B_{12} supplementation is usually recommended in pure vegetarian diets.

Why then do Hindu vegetarians who eat no animal products at all not have vitamin B_{12} deficiency problems? Unintentional contamination with animal products is probably the explanation. Parts of insects or their eggs or soil microorganisms get into the foods during growth or storage. Insects are not only a source of animal protein, but of vitamins such as B_{12} as well. Contamination is not just a problem in places like India, however. Keeping food 100 percent pure is virtually impossible, and the health regulations set by the Food

The Commonsense Guide to Good Eating

and Drug Administration in this country allow a certain amount of "filth" in foods. This unintentional "fortification" may not be harmful to your health, but the thought of insects or rodent hairs ground up in your bread isn't very appealing, is it?

Also of concern is a recently published report suggesting that high doses of vitamin C (0.5 gram or more) popularly used as a home remedy against the common cold, may destroy substantial amounts of vitamin B_{12}.

Riboflavin

Though intestinal bacteria probably manufacture small amounts of riboflavin, milk supplies about 43 percent of all the riboflavin consumed by most Americans. Eggs are also a good source of this vitamin. If dairy products and eggs are excluded from your diet, you will need to eat liberal amounts of leafy vegetables, asparagus, broccoli, okra, winter squash, and dried beans or peas to meet your daily requirements. Fortunately, riboflavin is relatively stable in heat and only slightly soluble in cooking water. Thus, excessive losses of this vitamin during ordinary cooking are minimized.

Calcium

A large serving of about one cup of greens such as collards, kale, turnip, and mustard provides as much calcium as one cup of milk. Cabbage, broccoli, and cauliflower will contribute lesser amounts of calcium but more than most other vegetables. Other plant sources which are moderate-to-good sources of calcium include: legumes, particularly soybeans; some nuts, particularly almonds; and dried fruits. It must be remembered, however, that occasional use of these foods cannot be counted on to replace the calcium and riboflavin of milk.

Iron

Excluding meat and shellfish, the following are good sources of iron—in decreasing order of excellence: egg yolk, dried beans and other legumes, dried fruits, nuts, green leafy vegetables, whole-grain and enriched cereals and cereal products, and dark molasses. Milk is a poor source of iron.

Zinc

Zinc is minimally present in fruits, vegetables, and refined foods. Oysters are an unusually rich source. Whole grains are your best bet, followed by dry legumes and nuts.

Vitamin D

A city-dwelling vegetarian who avoids milk products will often require a vitamin D supplement. Egg yolks, fortified milk, fish oils, and liver are the usual sources of this nutrient. Sunshine acting on the skin causes formation of vitamin D in the body and is usually sufficient for an adult who spends a good deal of time outside. Supplementation is usually recommended for infants, children, and pregnant women.

Iodine, niacin, thiamin, vitamins A and D

A recent Health and Nutrition Survey in the United States showed various segments of our population to be at risk for deficiencies of these nutrients. The survey and its findings is discussed under the various nutrients in the Appendix in The Whys and Wherefores of Vitamins and Minerals.

The most important safeguard for vegetarians is variety in the diet. The greatest risk comes from undue reliance on a single plant food source. Legumes, particularly soybeans, are rich in protein, B-vitamins, and iron. Grains are good sources of carbohydrates, proteins, thiamin, iron, and trace minerals. Nuts and other seeds contribute fat, protein, B-vitamins, and iron. Dark green, leafy vegetables are sources of calcium, riboflavin, and carotene — a precursor of vitamin A — and should be used liberally by pure vegetarians.

Deficiencies are harmful to us all, but they are especially dangerous when the body is in a growth period. A small but significant number of cases with severe deficiencies have already been reported where dairy products have been excluded from the diet. If irreversible damage to a child's health and body is to be avoided, we must provide the necessary dietary information required to ensure an adequate diet without unduly compromising the parents' beliefs. Otherwise, their offspring may be lost to medical surveillance forever.

Also keep in mind that nutritional requirements are greatly accentuated by illness. There is excessive breakdown of body protein, as well as a depletion of other vital nutrients, during febrile illnesses, after injuries, burns, or surgery.

Types of Vegetarianism

You might be interested in the different kinds of vegetarians there are:
- Lacto-vegetarians use dairy products such as milk, cheese, and butter.
- Lacto-ovo-vegetarians also include eggs in their diet.
- Macrobiotics ("longevity") is a Zen ("meditation") dietary system, originated by a man named Georges Ohsawa, that strives for a progressively limited diet according to spiritual development. The ultimate objective is a diet of brown rice alone. A very dangerous objective, we might add.
- Mono-vegetarians eat only one food, such as brown rice or soybeans. A *most undesirable goal*.

- Natural vegetarians will not eat refined or processed foods, such as sugar or bleached flour. Some will eat only raw, uncooked foods.
- Pure vegetarians only use grains, legumes, nuts, fruits, and vegetables. Some pure vegetarians will not eat honey, but others will.
- Vegans are pure vegetarians who, for ethical reasons, refrain from using any animal products of any kind, even leather. Vegans often refuse vaccinations because they are prepared from animal cultures.

Actually, the lacto-ovo-vegetarian diet does not differ markedly from the average American diet. The main difference is that it replaces meat with a variety of legumes, meat analogs, cereals, and nuts and more generous intakes of milk and milk products and some eggs. In practice, the nutritional composition of this type of diet is strengthened by the variety of foods which replace the meat. Additionally, the reduction of saturated fats and cholesterol, the increase in fiber, and the apparent cholesterol-lowering effect of leguminous seeds all seem to offer health advantages. It is also of interest that vegetarians usually weigh less—more closely approaching their "ideal" weight—than meat eaters. This might be a fact worth remembering for those with excess weight.

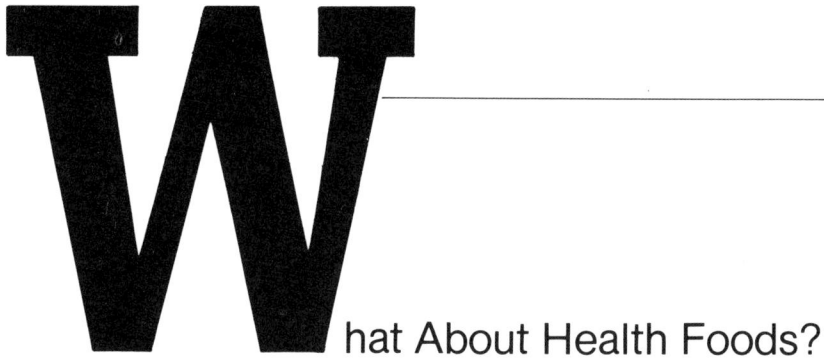

What About Health Foods?

The Real Concerns, Plus Some Questions and Answers

Over the last few years, health food stores have sprung up in large and small cities throughout the country. Like all businesses, some are good and some are bad. Without question, some stores offer overpriced products with supposedly near magic properties. Also without question, many people go to such stores hoping to find foods with supernatural powers capable of curing or warding off almost every ailment known to mankind from the common cold to cancer. To brand all health food store owners as charlatans, and all their customers as fanatics would, however, be an insult to their integrity and to our own intelligence. So let's get down to the issues that are of concern to most health food enthusiasts.

Organically Grown Foods

In general, the term *organic food* refers to foods that have been grown without the use of chemical pesticides or herbicides, where the fertilization of the soil has been done with natural composting rather than manufactured fertilizers, and where the handling of the product following its production has been without the use of any type of food additive.

People choose these products for a variety of reasons. Some feel that naturally fertilized foods are more nutritious than commercially fertilized products, that chemical pest controls and additives are dangerous to your health, and that organic farming is nonpolluting. Natural food producers believe that natural fertilizer builds up the soil, while they believe that chemical fertilizer wears the soil out, making it necessary to use more and more chemical fertilizer each year. There is also a general trend to the more "natural" way of doing things.

There is no scientific evidence that organically grown foods are any more or less nutritious than foods grown using commercial fertilizers. The soil and growing plant reduce all fertilizers to inorganic components before using the nutrients. Though slight variations in the nutritive value of crops can be related to the soil, most nutrients — except minerals — are synthesized by the plant, not absorbed from the soil. Fertilization primarily affects the quantity of the crop rather than the quality. The nutritive value of a food is primarily dependent on genetic determinants, the minerals that are found in the soil (commercial fertilizers are often designed to compensate for the lack of minerals in certain soils), the plants access to sunlight, and the maturity of the crops at harvest.

Everyone is entitled to believe what he or she wants, however, and if people choose to buy one product over another because they feel the one to be the more nutritious, then that's their business. What should be of concern to us all, however, is whether customers are actually getting what they think they are paying for. Many chemically fertilized products have been found to be purposely mislabeled "organically grown." Misrepresentation is against the law, and it can lead to serious health damage to its victims.

To many natural food eaters, doing things naturally helps them to see people's interrelationship with nature and to feel a part of nature. Many of these people are members of an ecological movement to use and reuse things, recycling items as nature does through decomposition. Many of them also believe that modern medicine is centered too much around curative medicine instead of preventive medicine. Herbal medicine uses herbs and natural foods, and it tends to be more preventive in intent than curative.

Anyone desiring to take up organic gardening on their own should be warned of the dangers of using fertilizers of animal or human origin. These can contain gastrointestinal parasites, and disease becomes a possibility. A little self-education about this potential problem is advised.

Chemical Pesticides

Are chemical pesticides necessary? Where practical, natural predators such as wasps and praying mantises may be used to control certain pests. Such an approach unfortunately is not adequate presently for the commercial production of enough food to meet the needs of this country and to contribute to the alleviation of world food problems.

Over the years, a number of innovative nonchemical pesticides have proven effective, but usually chemical pesticides have proven to be cheaper and more rapidly applied. One wonders, however, that if our great scientific know-how was forced to focus on the problem perhaps alternative means would be developed. While complete elimination of chemical pesticides and of pesticide residues in food is probably not practical, the safety of those used should be clearly established.

What About Health Foods?

Are chemical pesticides dangerous to our health? There has been and will, no doubt, continue to be considerable debate over this question. The Food and Drug Administration as well as the Department of Agriculture and the Environmental Protection Agency are authorized to conduct a continuing series of programs to make sure that pesticides are not used in such a way that they leave "poisonous" residues, and to see that pesticides that can't be used without leaving illegal residues are not used at all. Products are to be monitored, and those found to contain levels of pesticides above that permitted by regulation are supposed to be seized and taken off the market. But this still doesn't answer the question of whether pesticides are dangerous to our health, does it? Let's look at some of the factors involved.

Once a pesticide is certified for use, the Food and Drug Administration (FDA) sets the amount of residue allowed ("tolerance") to remain on vegetables, fruits, meats, and other foods. In setting these tolerances, the FDA attempts to establish a level that will protect the general public from the harm of poisonous residues. How is this tolerance figure arrived at? Primarily by observing what the chemicals do to animals and then setting the level considerably below that which causes observable damage to the animals. This raises a number of issues and problems.

What is "poisonous"? What do we mean by "observable" damage? The dictionary defines *poisonous* as "having the properties or effect of poison"; that is, "a substance that through its chemical action usually kills, injures, or impairs an organism." Obviously, sudden illness or death is readily "observable," but what about less immediate, more long-term injuries or impairments such as fewer and less healthy babies? And what about the fact that you are probably taking in many chemicals, not just the one being tested, by way of other foods, polluted air and water, cigarette smoke, drugs, etc.?

Though an attempt is made to adjust tolerances to take into consideration multiple chemical ingestions, many question the safety of these tolerances. Additionally, the FDA does not routinely consider indications that a pesticide may cause genetic changes. Then, too, consider the problem of trying to monitor 900 separate pesticide chemicals, which are combined into 45,000 different pesticide products, one-half of which are used in and around the home.

It is also of concern that pesticides often find their way to places far removed from the source of their original application, carried to the most remote corners of the world by wind, river, and sea. For example, scientists exploring Antarctica have found traces of DDT on a continent where it has never been used and where, in fact, few men have ever been.

Critics of widespread indiscriminate use of pesticides point out that chemicals that can kill insects and plant pests can also have an effect on animals and humans and should be more carefully controlled. The safety of the tolerance levels should be clearly established, and then adherence to the levels should be *strictly* enforced. However, Rachel Carson in her book *Silent Spring* suggests that the very idea of setting a tolerance for chemicals known to be harmful is questionable — "deliberately poisoning our food, then policing the result."

Food Additives

By and large, food additives can be divided into six general classes: 1) nutrient supplements — composed of vitamins or minerals and added to some foods to improve their nutritive value; 2) flavoring agents — added to some foods to make them more palatable; 3) preservatives — includes a vast variety of substances that are added to some foods which would otherwise fall prey to spoilage organisms or undergo undesirable chemical changes before being consumed; 4) emulsifiers — often used in bakery goods to improve the volume and fineness of grain and in dairy products to maintain a smooth, freely flowing product; 5) stabilizers and thickeners — used for maintenance of smooth texture and to give body to certain foods; 6) agents to control acidity or alkalinity — the production of quality baked goods, soft drinks, and confectioneries depends upon the availability of acids, alkalies, and buffers.

Other additives are used to mature and bleach flour, retain moisture, color, sterilize, harden, dry, leaven, and to carry out a number of other functions. The propellant for food in pressurized cans is considered a food additive. One wonders if the insects, rodent droppings, mold, and other debris found in food shouldn't be considered another class of additives!

The Food and Drug Administration (FDA) is responsible for the safety of all food additives and it is allowed to place the burden of proof on the manufacturer of the additives or food product. There are many, including some FDA scientists, who question the thoroughness of the safety tests and the decisions being made on the basis of the data. Such divided opinion about the safety of a number of additives casts a shadow of doubt over the GRAS ("generally recognized as safe") list which has been developed.

One of the more disturbing aspects of this debate over the safety of food additives is that the public is not given the opportunity to make a choice about whether or not to purchase foods containing additives because many — nearly 500 — ingredients do not have to be listed on labels. In fact, labeling standards are so inconsistent that a chemical may have to be listed as an ingredient of one food and not of another. MSG, for example, must be noted on soup labels but not on mayonnaise or salad dressing labels. Thus, by looking at the label you have no way of knowing whether or not the additive is present. And this is the situation at a time when the public's right to give their "informed consent" after having the possible risks and benefits explained is proclaimed so loudly!

What About Health Foods?

Can we do without food additives? Probably not entirely, but many that were used in the past for valid reasons could probably be eliminated now. For example, in this day of mass food production and rapid refrigerated transport systems, spoilage is not the problem that it was once. Some additives whose inclusion was approved when conditions were less favorable could probably be eliminated. Better sanitary conditions during processing could eliminate others.

On the other hand, if using certain additives to minimize spoilage and extend shelf-life helps keep food production costs down, this could benefit both industry and the consumer. Judging from current food prices, however, one has difficulty in believing that any of these savings are being passed along to the public.

About three-fifths of the food additives used are artificial flavors and colors, emulsifiers, stabilizers, and thickeners whose main purpose is to make foods more attractive. This function may well be challenged. Unfortunately, however, Madison Avenue and the whole food industry has done a good job of convincing people of the merits of today's conveniently packaged and pleasingly colored foods. A re-education program is in order. Until then, if these additives make nutritious foods look and taste appealing and without them such foods would not find wide acceptance, they may be as beneficial as the preservatives, antioxidants, leaveners, anti-staleness, and mold-retarding agents that help protect the consumer from bacteria and toxins. Certainly, sophisticated use of chemistry will be needed to give things like soy protein isolate, fish meal, and algae acceptable tastes and textures.

At any rate, food labels ought to name all ingredients so that those concerned about product safety and those who have allergic or other medical problems can make intelligent decisions. Some opponents of food additives have suggested that labels ought to carry a warning about possible health hazards. Experience with the impact of the labeling of poisonous household substances on the incidence of poisoning would suggest that this would probably not affect consumption, however.

Possible forces working against the effectiveness of poison labeling that might have some relevance to nutritional labeling are: attractive container and advertising on side of product that faces customer when item is on display, whereas warning is on back of item without embellishment (there is nothing on the front of the item to make the customer *want* to turn to the back label); price tag often placed over warning; parents don't read label and children can't read label; intensive educational programs were not mounted.

Why Your Child is Hyperactive, is a recent book by Dr. Ben F. Feingold, in which he outlines his theory that hyperactivity in children is aggravated by synthetic colors and flavors and salicylates found in hundreds of U.S. food products. This book has had an alarming effect on the many thousands of parents of hyperactive children. Many critics and two separate studies done by medical teams to determine the scientific validity of Feingold's assumptions have found no solid scientific evidence for support of this theory. The controversy is likely to rage until definite proof can be established or the contention disproved.

Hyperactivity is a peculiarly American affliction. Its increase is a major concern but its cure should not be haphazard and experimental, particularly when removal of the supposedly offending agents could produce a totally deficient diet in the inexperienced family. Parents with hyperactive children should disregard the furor of eliminating these additives — an almost impossible task — for the present.

Availability of Certain Products

It is a sad commentary on our food supply system that in many towns, the health food store is the only place you can find items such as soybeans, bean sprouts, cracked wheat, rye flour, and, in many instances, even whole wheat flour. It is also likely to be the only place where you can find cheese without artificial coloring added or a selection of products without preservatives or other additives. How often have you eaten or seen the natural white cheddar cheese?

Some Questions and Answers

Are brown eggs better for you than white ones?
And how about fertile eggs versus regular eggs?

The nutritive value of an egg is not related to the color of the shell or to whether the egg is fertile or not. One danger of fertile eggs is that they spoil much more rapidly than nonfertile ones. Egg color is determined by the breed of the hen.

How do blackstrap molasses, sugar, and honey compare nutritionally?

Blackstrap molasses contains calcium, iron, and most of the B vitamins and is slightly lower in calories than sugar and honey. Dark brown sugar retains some of the molasses from which purified sugar crystals are separated and, thus, contains a small amount of the minerals — but not the vitamins — found in molasses. White sugar is a source of nothing but calories! Honey contains some vitamins, but otherwise is little different from brown sugar.

What About Health Foods?

How does white flour compare with whole wheat flour?
When white flour products are enriched, they are equal or better sources of thiamine, riboflavin, niacin, and iron than whole wheat flour. Not all the nutrients removed in the milling process are returned, however, and thus whole wheat flour contains a wider array of nutrients than white flour, even when the latter is enriched. Whole grain products are also a good source of roughage.

Are untreated vegetable oils preferable to commercial vegetable oils?
Untreated vegetable oils have been cold-pressed and bottled with no additives or preservatives. They are, therefore, more perishable. Proper storage in a cool, dry place will help prevent them from becoming rancid, however.

What is lecithin?
Lecithin is a fatlike substance found widely in foods and also synthesized by the body. Despite various claims, there is no proof that lecithin can reduce blood cholesterol levels. Nor does it have any magical weight-reducing properties, regardless of what other substance it is mixed with.

Will gelatin strengthen my fingernails?
Despite its animal origin, gelatin is an incomplete protein; it does not contain all the amino acids needed for growth, repair, and maintenance. There are differences of scientific opinion as to whether protein in any form improves fingernails.

Will vitamin A cure acne?
The use of vitamin A in the treatment of acne has been largely one of hit and miss. At any rate, it should be attempted only under the supervision of a physician. Remember, vitamin A can be toxic when taken in large doses for prolonged periods of time.

What are the benefits to be derived from using brewer's yeast?
Brewer's yeast is a good source of B vitamins, amino acids, and minerals and could be used as a source of these nutrients should your diet be deficient in these areas. A tablespoon of powdered brewer's yeast contains 27 calories.

Should I restrict my intake of caffeine?
It depends upon how you feel. Are you restless? Do you have insomnia? Is your heart rate rapid and sometimes irregular? Even young people can suffer from caffeine binges. It could be those daily half-dozen soft drinks or

The Commonsense Guide to Good Eating

perhaps even that pain-relieving drug you are taking on special occasions.

All cola beverages contain caffeine. The Food and Drug Administration permits the use of caffeine in these beverages up to 1.2 grains (72 mg) per 12 ounce bottle (6 mg/oz.). Low-calorie drinks are allowed only half (3 mg/oz.) as much caffeine.

The amount of caffeine found in some cola beverages, on a per fluid ounce basis, is as follows: Coca-Cola, 4.6 mg; Pepsi-Cola, 3 mg; and Royal Crown Cola, 3.5 mg.

The caffeine content of an average cup of coffee, prepared from 15 to 17 grams of coffee and averaging 5 fluid ounces, would be approximately 18 mg/fl.oz. Strong tea would contain the same amount of caffeine, although average tea would approximate 12 to 15 mg/fl.oz. Cocoa contains about 6 mg per ounce. Popular pain-relieving drugs often contain 30 mg or more of caffeine. Last but not least, on that long trip, don't forget that caffeine is a notorious diuretic.

Incidentally, despite all the recent studies, there is still no proof that there is a direct relationship between drinking coffee and heart attacks. If, indeed, it turns out that heavy coffee drinkers suffer more heart attacks than others, it may be that coffee drinking is just part of the heart attack-prone person's personality traits. There still may not be a chemical relationship between the two. There is sufficient controversy about this point, however, that many persons have switched to decaffinated coffee "just to be on the safe side."

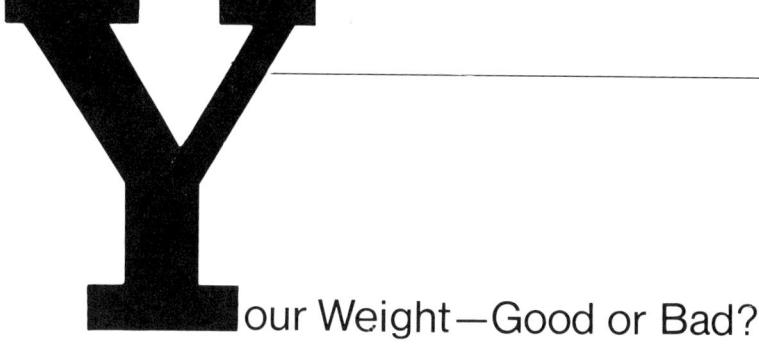our Weight—Good or Bad?

Twelve Questions and Answers About Your Weight

How accurate are those height-weight charts?
Most height-weight charts describe the "average" person in this country. Since many physicians agree that obesity (excessive fatness) is one of our leading health problems today, "average" weight should not be confused with "ideal" or "desirable" weight.

What then is your ideal or desirable weight? It is the pounds you weigh when there is no excess body *fat* present. Table 5 will give you a reasonable estimate of the weight that might be appropriate for your height and body build. You will notice that the weight allowances are much lower than in the charts you so often run across, and that age has not been used as one of the determining factors. Age is not really a consideration except during active growth periods; it is the relationship of weight to height and bone and muscle that is critical in evaluating your weight.

Not everyone who is heavy is harboring excess fat; the extra weight could be owing to a heavy bone structure and very developed muscle tissue. Our concern is with excess body fat, however, and this presents a problem because whereas weight is easily measured, fatness is not.

If scales give only a reading of overall weight, without any real indication of how much of that weight is excess fat, how can I tell if I'm too fat?
Strip and then take a good long look at yourself in the mirror. If you're not happy with what you see, or if you can "pinch" more than one inch of skin and underlying tissue over your ribs, you are probably carrying excess fat.

One way that doctors cope with this problem of measuring fat is through the use of a caliper, an instrument that can be adjusted to determine thickness. As a large proportion of body fat is carried under the skin, your pinch is similar to the measurement the doctor makes with the caliper.

The Commonsense Guide to Good Eating

TABLE 5
HEIGHT/WEIGHT CHART[1]

Height	"Desirable"[2]			"Ideal"[3]		
	Small Frame	Medium Frame	Large Frame	Small Frame	Medium Frame	Large Frame
Women						
4'8"	88- 94	92-103	100-115	80- 85	83- 93	90-104
9	90- 97	94-106	102-118	81- 88	85- 96	92-107
10	92-100	97-109	105-121	83- 90	88- 99	95-109
11	95-103	100-112	108-124	86- 93	90-101	98-112
5'0"	98-106	103-115	111-127	89- 96	93-104	100-115
1	101-109	106-118	114-130	91- 99	96-107	103-117
2	104-112	109-122	117-134	94-101	99-110	105-121
3	107-115	112-126	121-138	97-104	101-114	109-125
4	110-119	116-131	125-142	99-108	105-118	113-128
5	114-123	120-135	129-146	103-111	108-122	117-132
6	118-127	124-139	133-150	107-115	112-126	120-135
7	122-131	128-143	137-154	110-118	116-129	123-139
8	126-136	132-147	141-157	114-123	119-133	127-142
9	130-140	136-151	145-164	117-126	123-136	131-148
10	134-144	140-155	149-169	121-130	126-140	135-153
11	138-148	144-159	153-174	125-134	130-145	138-157
6'0"	142-152	149-163	157-179	128-137	135-147	142-162
Men						
5'0"	101-109	107-117	115-130	91- 99	97-106	104-117
1	104-112	110-121	118-133	94-101	99-109	107-120
2	107-115	113-125	121-136	97-104	102-113	109-123
3	110-118	116-128	124-140	99-107	105-116	112-126
4	113-121	119-131	127-144	102-109	108-118	115-130
5	116-125	122-135	130-148	105-113	110-122	117-134
6	120-129	126-139	134-153	108-117	114-126	121-138
7	124-133	130-144	139-158	112-120	117-130	126-143
8	128-137	134-148	143-162	116-124	121-134	129-146
9	132-142	138-152	147-166	119-128	125-137	133-150
10	136-146	142-157	151-171	123-132	128-142	136-154
11	140-150	146-162	156-176	126-135	132-146	141-159
6'0"	144-154	150-167	160-181	130-139	135-151	144-163
1	148-158	154-172	165-186	134-143	139-155	149-168
2	152-162	159-177	170-191	137-146	144-160	153-172
3	156-167	164-182	174-196	141-151	148-164	157-177
4	160-171	169-187	178-201	144-154	153-169	161-181

[1] Heights and weights are without clothing.
[2] Adapted from Metropolitan Life Insurance Company Tables which are based on weights associated with the lowest mortality.
[3] Ten percent less than "Desirable" weights. This weight level is considered by many physicians to be your healthiest weight. This is especially true for persons with diabetes.
Note: There is no easy, reliable way to measure body "frame" though many methods such as measuring wrist size have been proposed. The notion of differences in frame size is probably more harmful than helpful, as many persons try to justify their excess weight with the excuse that they have "a large frame."

Your Weight—Good or Bad?

With increasing age, there tends to be a concentration of fatty tissue over the abdomen, so a side view of yourself in the mirror is advisable. Also, it's not a bad idea to keep in mind that most people are at their best weight at about age twenty years. If you are over twenty and weigh much more than you did at that age, you are probably overweight. This assumes, of course, that you were not overweight at age twenty!

The words *overweight* and *obesity* are often used interchangeably. Most workers in the field of weight evaluation and regulation would not agree with this usage and would argue for a more precise definition of each word. Even among specialists, however, there is no agreement about how to define obesity. Some consider a person who is more than ten percent over his or her desirable weight to be obese; others set the limit at twenty percent; and still others use an even higher percentage.

In general, however, we can say that *overweight* refers to a body weight in excess of some standard, whereas *obesity* refers not just to weight but to one's state of "fatness."

Weight in excess of some standard—such as shown on "average" or "desirable" weight charts—does not tell us whether the weight is owing to fat, bone, muscle, or fluid. Thus, a football player may weigh more than weight charts would indicate as average or desirable and still not be obese. His overweight is likely to be the result of well-developed bone and muscle. On the other hand, a person may weigh within the desirable range, but still be carrying an excess of fat. This is why the pinch test described above is a valuable aid in evaluating your weight and degree of fatness.

Chances are, however, if you are ten percent above the weight identified as desirable for your height and body build, you are probably obese; that is, you are carrying around unhealthy fat. A twenty percent increase in your weight leaves little doubt about your condition.

It is estimated that up to forty percent of our population may be overweight, with about twenty percent of the population being more than twenty percent above their best weight.

It is clear that the great majority of obese—extremely overweight—children become obese adults. It is not clear, however, what are all factors involved in this relationship. Eating patterns are obviously one part of the problem, but researchers are showing that an overproduction of fat cells at an early age is also significant.

In studies done on rats, it was found that obesity in young rats was a result of too many fat cells, while obesity that started in adulthood was owing not to the addition of more fat cells but to an increase in the size of already existing fat cells. It also appears that there is no way to get rid of extra fat cells once they are formed; the best you can do is reduce them in size.

There is evidence that this animal observation also has relevance in human beings. Fat cells produced in early life hang around like sponges to increase in size the rest of your life. Since overweight is a problem for more than fifty percent of teenagers, the solution to an overweight problem should be considered early in one's life.

Other than improving my looks, is there any reason to shed excess fat?

Absolutely. Study after study confirms that excessive weight aggravates every conceivable ailment, from back aches to varicose veins, and that excessive fat accumulation actually lays the foundation for many diseases.

A fifty-year-old man who is fifty pounds overweight has about half the life expectancy of a man of the same age who is of normal weight! Statistics also show that the overweight person suffers more than the normal weight person from heart disease, gall bladder disease, diabetes, and many other disorders. Additionally, excess fat increases the dangers of complications when surgery is required or during pregnancy. Overweight people also complain of leg and back pain; our skeletal system is not designed to carry the burden of extra weight.

Of equal importance is the sad fact that it is very difficult for the overweight, especially the excessively overweight, person to live in a society which sets great store by slimness. For, despite the large number of overweight people in this country, the body look we seem to prefer is one of trimmer proportions. Thus, fat people often find themselves the subject of ridicule. It is especially difficult for the overweight youngster to cope with being made fun of by his classmates. This often is the beginning of a lasting psychological and personality problem.

Obesity that starts early in childhood is usually harder to cope with later in life than the creeping obesity of middle age. Persons who become obese as youths often view their shape as a shame, rather than as a medical problem. By the time they're older, many have developed feelings of inadequacy and have a history of repeated failures at weight control. These individuals have become conditioned to expect failure.

Obesity that creeps up as you age and become less active is less likely to be associated with psychological problems. Individuals with this maturity-onset problem often recognize the health hazards associated with their obese state, and see their condition as reversible provided they receive proper medical attention and support.

In both instances — early-onset and maturity-onset obesity — prevention is preferable to treatment!

The more excessive the overweight and the older the person, the greater is the likelihood of suffering from the health hazards associated with overweight.

Your Weight—Good or Bad?

Unfortunately, however, it is well documented that obese children run a great risk of remaining obese all their lives. It has been estimated that for obese children of age twelve, the odds against being normal-weight adults are four to one, and if weight loss is not accomplished by the end of adolescence, the odds rise to twenty-eight to one. Early attention to one's dietary habits and weight regulation is, thus, clearly called for and extremely important.

Is there anyone who is overweight that shouldn't go on a reducing diet?

Yes! There are some rare medical conditions where weight reduction may be contraindicated. Also, if a person doesn't have a serious commitment to lose weight and then maintain the weight loss, they will probably regain the weight. This yo-yo effect may be more harmful to their health than a steady state of overweight.

Individuals with diverticulitis, gout, tuberculosis, Addison's disease, ulcerative colitis, and regional ileitis may be advised not to undertake a rigid weight-loss program. It is unlikely that many people will fall into this group, but it is still one more reason why people should check with their doctor before going on a weight reduction campaign.

Also, it is felt by some that *broad* fluctuations in weight may actually give rise to higher cholesterol levels and chances of artery damage than a higher but more stable weight. Thus, weight reduction should be only part of the obese person's goal—maintenance of the weight loss should be the other part of the goal.

Other important considerations are: emotional stability; circumstances in home, school, or office that may make it impossible to change eating and/or activity patterns; and growth patterns. Great care must be taken during periods of rapid bone growth to make sure that nutritional deficiencies don't occur.

How serious a problem is underweight?

Underweight may or may not be serious, depending on the degree a person is underweight and the age at which it occurs. Provided that the condition is not accompanied by a lack of protein, vitamins, or minerals, there are times when it is advantageous to be somewhat underweight. This is true for middle-aged or older persons, especially if they have any tendency toward diabetes, high blood pressure, heart trouble, or kidney disease. Severe underweight is almost sure to be a disadvantage, regardless of age, but is especially serious during active growth periods.

How thin is too thin?

If you are more than seven to ten percent below the ideal weight for your height and body build, you may be functioning at a lower energy level than you should. A tendency to chill and fatigue easily and to be susceptible to infection are common. Medical evaluation of your health status is called for.

Any evaluation of one's weight must take into account hereditary influences, general health, quantity and quality of energy intake in the form of food, and energy output in the form of exercise or "nervous energy." However, since many diseases have weight loss as one of their symptoms, sudden or excessive weight loss should be brought to the attention of your physician.

What is anorexia nervosa?

Anorexia means nothing more than a loss of appetite; this is a relatively common symptom of anxiety. Anorexia nervosa, however, is a condition marked by loss of appetite with loss of weight, accompanied by marked neurotic or psychotic symptoms.

The tie between food and one's state of mind is a strong one, dating back to early infancy. For the infant, the nursing or feeding process is more than just a way of gaining food; it is also a social and emotional experience with reactions of pleasure or pain, satisfaction or frustration, acceptance or rejection. Food may, thus, become identified with unconscious meanings that are far removed from the original concept of just eating. It may become a physical equivalent of love and acceptance, and an emotionally deprived youngster or adult may express his or her frustration in unconscious self-starvation. The condition may be precipitated by a relatively small criticism or confrontation with imperfection, such as being called fat or being unable to achieve in some athletic endeavor. Patients with anorexia nervosa present difficult problems both psychologically and nutritionally and their management is seldom easy.

Most cases of anorexia nervosa develop between puberty and the thirties, usually in unmarried women though at times marriage may be the precipitating factor. The person will often continue her usual life pattern, claiming all the while that she is in no way suffering from the self-imposed starvation. Menstrual periods disappear as the person's condition worsens. Anorexia nervosa requires expert and constant medical attention until corrected, or else irreparable psychological and nutritional deficits may remain.

How is weight regulated?

Weight maintenance, weight loss, weight gain — it's all a matter of calories:
- Caloric intake *equal* to activity and growth requirements = Weight *maintenance*

To maintain your weight, your caloric intake must not exceed your body's requirements. These requirements vary depending on how active you are and whether your body is undergoing unusual stress such as a growth spurt, pregnancy, or recovery from illness. The greater the body's requirement,

Your Weight—Good or Bad?

whether it is energy needed for exercise or for growth, the greater the caloric intake requirement. Most people overestimate their energy expenditures.
- Caloric intake *less* than activity and growth requirements = Weight *loss*

To lose weight, you must take in fewer calories than you require to maintain your weight. The more calories you eliminate, either through increased physical activity or by calorie elimination, the faster the weight loss.
- Caloric intake in *excess* of activity and growth requirement = Weight *gain*

To gain weight, your caloric intake must exceed that required for weight maintenance. Calories available for weight gain can be obtained through reduction of energy expenditure or by calorie addition.

Because of the magnitude and complexity of the problem, how to lose weight is dealt with in a separate chapter, "I'm Overweight! Now What?"

How many calories do I need?

In general, your body requires about fifteen calories a pound to keep you walking, breathing, at the proper body temperature, minimally active, and at a constant weight. We like to refer to this basic caloric requirement as your "maintenance level."

If you take in more calories than is required for your maintenance level, you will gain weight. If you take in fewer calories than is required for your maintenance level, you will lose weight.

If you are extremely inactive, you may require only twelve calories a pound for proper body and weight maintenance. A person actively growing or involved in a strenuous physical training program may require as many as twenty or twenty-five calories a pound for maintenance.

To calculate how many calories you require, you need to decide whether you are, in general, inactive or minimally, moderately, or highly active. Then, multiply your "ideal" or "desirable" weight by the number of calories needed to maintain your activity level. This will tell you how many calories you need each day to maintain your proper weight. Table 6 may be helpful.

How can I gain weight?

Increase your food intake by 500 calories a day above maintenance level, excercise lightly but regularly, and reduce tenseness by getting extra rest and relaxation. Avoid filling foods that contain few calories, such as clear soups.

To gain weight, you need first to rule out any possibility of illness. Even "nerves" can thwart your attempt to put on weight, so see your doctor and have a good check-up.

If your physician gives you a clean bill of health and doesn't feel that you are genetically predisposed to being thin you are ready to start your gain-weight program.

The Commonsense Guide to Good Eating

TABLE 6
CALORIES REQUIRED DAILY TO MAINTAIN NORMAL BODY FUNCTIONS

	Calories Required Daily to Maintain Normal Body Functions and Weight If You Are:			
Ideal or Desirable Weight	Inactive (12 cals/pound)	Minimally Active (15 cals/pound)	Moderately Active (20 cals/pound)	Highly Active (25 cals/pound)
100	1200	1500	2000	2500
110	1320	1650	2200	2750
120	1440	1800	2400	3000
130	1560	1950	2600	3250
140	1680	2100	2800	3500
150	1800	2250	3000	3750
160	1920	2400	3200	4000
170	2040	2550	3400	4250
180	2160	2700	3600	4500
190	2280	2850	3800	4750
200	2400	3000	4000	5000

To gain weight, you must take in more calories in food than your body uses in keeping you walking, breathing, and in good general repair. If you consume 500 calories a day every day in excess of what your body needs, you will gain about a pound a week — 500 calories/day x 7 days = 3,500 calories = 1 pound.

High-calorie foods can be added to your regular meals and/or they can be eaten as midmorning, midafternoon, or as bedtime snacks. If your appetite is poor, you will probably find that many small meals are easier to cope with than a few large meals. It may also be necessary to judge your need for food intake by the clock rather than by whether or not you feel hungry.

Exercise should not be shunned even though it obviously uses up calories. Exercise will not make you hungry, but it will tone and firm your muscles and contribute to a sense of general well-being which may make you more relaxed and thus more responsive to food stimuli. Besides, you will want to increase your weight by better muscular development and not through the addition of body fat alone.

How can I increase my caloric intake by 500 calories?

The extra calories don't need to be eaten all at one time. Spread them out over the day. Combinations of high-calorie but nonbulky foods are the best if your appetite is small.

For example, add eggs, brewer's yeast (make sure to buy one of the less bitter-tasting brands), sugar, honey or molasses, and vanilla to milk to yield eggnog, or enrich plain cold milk with cream or powdered milk. Add wheat germ to your regular cereal, scramble eggs in margarine or oil rather than eating them poached. Try cheese toast rather than plain bread. Cook meat in rich sauces or serve margarine or sauces with vegetables.

The richest source of calories is fat—more than twice the calories than in protein or carbohydrates—but you will want to try to control the amount and kind of fat in your diet. No more than thirty-five percent of your total daily calories should come from all kinds of fats. Saturated fats should be limited to ten percent of your allowance. Unfortunately, it may be impossible to both increase your daily caloric intake by 500 calories and to limit your fat intake. However, since such a diet would be necessary for a limited period of time, it is probably safe to deviate from the usual rules temporarily.

It will be worth your while to learn which foods are high in calories and which are not. For example, one tablespoon of peanut butter has the same number of calories as does four cups of cabbage! Refer to the chapters on Food Selection and Diet Plans for additional examples.

I'm underweight and have no real interest in food. Is there anything I can take to improve my appetite?

If your diet has been deficient in nutrients in addition to providing an inadequate calorie supply, taking a vitamin-mineral pill once a day may in general improve how you feel and thus stimulate your appetite.

Diets that are calorie deficient are often also lacking in an adequate supply of vitamins, minerals, and protein. One very common cause for a lack of vitality in young women is anemia due to iron deficiency. During a woman's reproductive years, she requires about twice as much iron as a man. This is owing to iron losses during menstrual periods and losses to the baby when pregnant or nursing. It is especially important that individuals with the above latter conditions be under the care and supervision of their physician.

It is well known that during periods of rapid growth, the body is especially vulnerable to injury from inadequate nutrition. Considering that your growth in height during the adolescent growth spurt proceeds more rapidly than at any time since infancy, it is easy to see why you should take care to meet your need for vitamins, minerals, and protein.

A word of caution about dietary supplements. Just because a little is good, a lot is not necessarily better. Certain vitamins, especially vitamins A and D, can be dangerous in high doses for a prolonged period of time. This is true for some minerals as well, especially iron. The chapter on Food Selection will help you make safe choices.

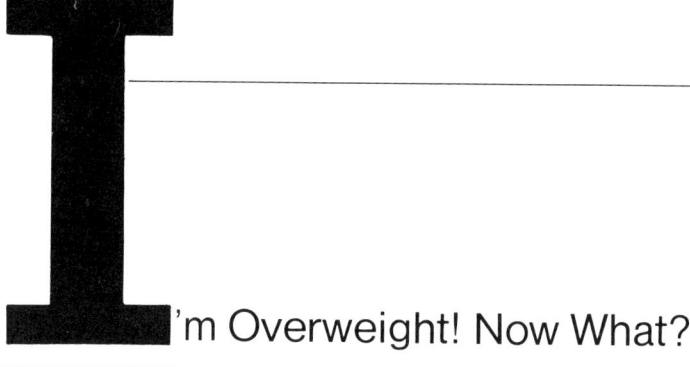'm Overweight! Now What?

Causes and Treatment
Plus Some Questions and Answers

Almost every new magazine brings with it a so-called new way to lose weight. Contrary to all claims for "miracle" diets, however, current scientific evidence points to only one way to lose weight: take in fewer calories in food than you use up in energy.

Everything you do, including sleeping, burns up a certain number of calories. Likewise, almost every food and drink that you take in adds calories of energy for your use or storage. The trick to dieting is to learn to regulate this input-output relationship. To assist you in this endeavor, we suggest that you start a "diet diary." This, plus seven steps to safe and effective dieting, will be explained in detail later on in this chapter. First, however, let's look at some of the factors involved in weight gains and some general approaches toward weight regulation.

What triggers obesity?

Though heredity may make a person more susceptible to unwanted fat storage, it still takes an imbalance between food intake and energy output to result in obesity.

When both parents are obese, the likelihood of the child also being obese is very high—eighty percent. When one parent is obese, the chance of the child being obese drops to forty percent. When neither parent is obese, the possibility of childhood obesity drops to only eight to nine percent.

Does this necessarily mean that the obesity is inherited? No. Home environment also plays a major role. If parents are inactive and tend to overeat, their children are likely to be inactive and overeat.

There is evidence, however, that genetic factors (heredity) do contribute to obesity. Much research remains to be done, though, before all the factors involved—and their relative significance—are identified and weighed.

Distribution of fat cells also seems to be inherited. If a woman has fat thighs, even though she is not fat anywhere else, no amount of dieting, exercising, or massage is likely to bring her legs down to what she might consider ideal proportions.

Do obese people consume more calories than normal-weight people? Not necessarily. Obese individuals do seem to be much less active, however, thus burning up fewer calories than normal-weight individuals. It has been shown repeatedly that overweight—especially excessively overweight—people are much less active than others. And it's not just a matter of doing or not doing the same activities. Even if an overweight person and a desirable weight person both "go swimming" for the same amount of time, the overweight person will move around much less than his or her thinner companion.

Is it my glands?

Most probably not.

It is routine, good medical practice to check for possible endocrine disorders when evaluating the excessively overweight person. The chances of such disorders being responsible for obesity are, however, remote. Even when present, the correction of such problems makes weight control easier but usually will not change the need for caloric restriction and increased exercise.

When is obesity most likely to occur?

In women, excessive weight gain often occurs after the cessation of adolescent growth, during pregnancies, and after menopause.

It is easy to understand why these are particularly susceptible periods. When the rate of growth slows down at the end of adolescence, food habits must be altered to compensate for the reduced caloric needs. In addition, this is the age at which many women either take a sedentary office job and/or get married and set up housekeeping which often means less physical activity.

Pregnancy often takes its toll when the mother feels she must "eat for two," while at the same time she is decreasing her activity level. Those extra pounds don't just miraculously disappear after the baby is born. Breast feeding helps extra pounds disappear, though.

Menopause is another common time for weight gain among women. A decrease in the basal metabolic rate may be partially responsible, but changes in activity patterns in middle age, endocrine activity and perhaps psychological factors that affect eating and activity patterns may also be significant.

For men, there are no such clearly identifiable times when excessive weight gain is especially likely. The typical pattern of weight gain in men begins in the early twenties—again, when the adolescent growth spurt is over—and continues gradually through middle age. Athletes particularly are susceptible, for once they retire from amateur or professional sports, they often fail to cut down on their daily food and calorie intake with cessation of their strenuous activities.

What is the treatment for obesity?

The treatment for obesity is a complex affair because the causes of obesity are many, are overlapping, and often are not fully understood.

How much "over-fat" one is, and whether there are any physical or mental problems are important considerations. In general, however, treatment consists of setting a reasonable goal and then designing a diet that is compatible with the individual's physical condition, occupation, food preferences, cultural background, and food budget. The diet and the general health of the individual are enhanced by the adoption of a regular pattern of exercise.

The obese child presents special and difficult problems, for treatment involves treating the parents as well, since they control the eating and exercising patterns of their children to a great extent.

Appetite suppressants (diet pills) are sometimes used until the person learns to adjust to the new diet pattern. However, these should only be taken under the supervision of a physician. This will be discussed more thoroughly in a later question.

Techniques of behavior modification—described in the next question-answer—also offer real hope and help for changing eating habits. Tricks such as eating at only one place in one room, slowing the pace of eating, not engaging in any other activity—such as reading or watching television—while eating and avoiding the purchase of problematic foods are all surprisingly effective in avoiding eating patterns that contribute to weight problems.

In extreme cases of obesity, the person may be hospitalized and put on a "starvation" diet. This total fasting should never be undertaken without medical supervision.

In recent years, surgical treatment for severe cases of obesity has been used. This operation, in which part of the intestines is removed, is not without its complications and dangers, however. The procedure is, therefore, usually employed only in severe, life-threatening situations.

What is behavior modification and can it help me?

Behavior modification is a technique that can be used to identify where, when, and why you eat and then help you change the habits that may be contributing to your weight problem. Many people have found behavior modification to mean the difference between success and failure in their efforts to control their weight.

By and large, obese people respond more to external eating cues—sight or smell of food—than to internal cues—hunger pangs. In many cases, external cues may actually trigger internal cues. For example an external cue may *at first* have nothing to do with food—watching television, for instance—but later the cue may become so associated with food—eating while watching television or during the commercials—that the external cue (in this case, television) will actually trigger an internal response of hunger.

Thus, the person who eats while watching television in the living room, or while reading in his bedroom, or while talking on the phone in the office may actually come to associate not only the activity—but the environment where the activity takes place with eating!

Developing the habit of brushing one's teeth immediately after eating could become a deterrent to snacking between meals for the more determined and fastidious individual. Therefore, some of the things that behavior modification teaches us is that it is necessary to:
- Eat in only one room.
- Eat at only one place in that room.
- Do not engage in any other activity while eating.
- Brush your teeth immediately after eating.

Do crash or fad diets work?

There really are redeeming qualities to some fad and/or crash diets. There are drawbacks as well. If you know both sides of the story, however, you are in a better position to maximize the positive aspects and minimize those that are negative. The pros and cons stack up this way:

ADVANTAGES	DISADVANTAGES
You feel you're really doing something about your weight.	Crash diets are hard to live with; consequently they are rather quickly abandoned, leaving you feeling guilty.
Weight loss can be seen fairly rapidly.	
Limited food selection keeps you from having to worry so much about calories.	Weight usually reappears just as rapidly as it is lost once the diet is stopped because you haven't changed your normal eating habits.
	You aren't learning to live in "the real world."
Extreme low-carbohydrate diets sometimes reduce the feeling of hunger.	Some diets are extremely dangerous.

It is important to realize that persons who require small weight losses and persons who require large weight losses make up two different groups, and the guidelines for weight loss are quite different for each. In general, there

I'm Overweight! Now What?

are two separate and equally important phases of management. Phase 1 is the weight loss phase during which time the usual nutritional rules and usual eating habits must be abandoned. Phase 2 consists of the re-introduction of normal nutritional patterns.

It is possible to combine Phase 1 and Phase 2 in persons who require only a small weight loss. However, to ask the person who requires a large weight loss to conform to "normal" nutritional standards and to "live in the real world" is to ask for failure.

There is probably nothing seriously wrong with going on a reasonably balanced but low-calorie crash diet while you're all psyched up about your weight condition, but use the time before you get bored with the diet to learn something about the caloric and nutrient values of different foods. While dieting strenuously, remember to take daily a vitamin-mineral supplement.

The diets that are likely to be harmful are those that sharply curtail food selection or those that delete carbohydrates. When food selection is narrowed to but a few choices, chances are you won't get an adequate protein or vitamin-mineral supply. You can, of course, partially remedy this by taking a daily vitamin-mineral supplement, but if your protein intake is also inadequate a vitamin pill will not solve this problem. Protein supplements are also available, but not only are they expensive, they also add additional calories — so why not just get the protein from food in the first place; it's a lot more satisfying! A word of warning: the Federal Trade Commission says that protein supplements can be most dangerous for infants under one year of age and for older people with liver or kidney ailments, whose systems cannot handle the highly concentrated doses. Unfortunately, this warning does not appear on most packages.

Another problem with trying to meet your nutritional needs with pills is that nutritionists aren't really sure that we have knowledge about all of the nutrients that food contains. Only those vitamins and minerals identified thus far are available in pill form. Food could well contain other necessary nutrients that scientists haven't discovered yet or for which the required amounts are not known.

Extremely low-carbohydrate diets present a possibly serious threat. Carbohydrates are necessary to prevent ketosis, a state wherein large quantities of ketones arise from a breakdown of fat. When the number of ketones in the blood displace the bicarbonate in the blood, the delicate acid-base balance of the blood is disturbed and acidosis develops. This is of critical importance to people with diabetes because, for them, ketosis can lead to coma and death if unchecked. Unfortunately, there are approximately 1.5 million people whose diabetic or pre-diabetic state has not been diagnosed and who may be adversely affected by such a diet. For the average healthy person, a diet which gets 50 to 100 grams of digestible carbohydrates, or at least fifteen percent of its energy from carbohydrates, will prevent ketosis. Diabetic diets are usually forty percent carbohydrates.

The Commonsense Guide to Good Eating

Carbohydrates are important for other reasons as well. They play a predominant role in the metabolism of the nervous system. Also of concern is the fact that diets low in carbohydrates and high in fat content load up your arteries with potentially harmful fat and cholesterol. Such diets, when taken over prolonged periods of time, greatly increase the likelihood of coronary artery disease. For more information on the relationship of diet to artery and heart disease, see the chapter on Atherosclerosis—Prevention Begins at an Early Age.

It should be noted, however, that ketogenic diets have been used medically for many years for the treatment of obesity as well as other disorders such as epilepsy. This is usually done under close medical supervision. Recently, ketogenic diets have become very popular, however, and many people have gone on those diets without medical consultation. It is not known how the majority of these people have fared.

One should also be wary of "eat kelp and grow thin" diets; they may be responsible for the development of hypothyroidism, or iodide goiter, in some people. Although most people can eat kelp without harm—it is nutritious and low in calories, and is a diet staple in Japan—it does contain a large amount of potassium iodide and has the potential to produce the above conditions. It is estimated that one to three precent of Americans have an underlying sensitivity to iodides and they would be particularly vulnerable to the kelp diet.

Is there any way to diet without feeling like I'm starving?

Spread your caloric allowance over the entire day. Many small meals or low-caloried snacks between major meals will ward off that feeling of hunger. Learn what foods are filling but low in calories. Keep a supply of fresh carrot, green pepper, and celery sticks on hand. You can eat two ribs of celery, two carrots, and one green pepper and you will have consumed only 100 calories. Drink chicken or beef bouillon between meals; it's only about seven calories a cup, but its salt content is high and therefore should not be abused. Some people find that a small number of sweets taken with a hot drink before a meal reduces their appetite—witness the boon in "reducing" candies.

Stay busy! Boredom is the major reason most people overeat. Try to stay out of the kitchen while food is cooking; the aroma and the urge to sneak a taste may be your undoing. Wash the dishes if this is your job, but get someone else to put away the food; the temptation to pick is an unnecessary complication in your efforts to lose weight.

Don't feel that you have to totally avoid foods containing fat. Fats are slower to leave the stomach than other foods and, thus, leave you feeling satisfied longer. Also, a small amount of fat is required for the absorption of the "fat-soluble" vitamins A, D, E, and K.

I'm Overweight! Now What?

What about using drugs to kill my appetite?

Any drug which alters brain function is potentially dangerous, and some are addictive. The few effective "diet pills" are available only by prescription; most, but not all, of those sold over-the-counter contain methyl cellulose which, though harmless, has shown little if any effect in promoting weight loss.

The correct way to use diet pills is as an aid in suppressing appetite while you go about the business of developing better eating patterns. Unfortunately, some people come to depend on the pills instead of using them to improve their dietary habits. This is, indeed, hazardous since long-term use of such a drug can produce many serious side-effects. Even more serious are those drugs that can make the body chemically dependent on them. To further complicate the picture is the fact that the longer you use these drugs, the less effective they become and, thus, the higher the dose that is required. Needless to say, this increases your likelihood of ill effects.

Diet pills should be taken ONLY when dieting under the supervision of a physician! Don't share your friend's supply.

Anorectics (drugs to reduce appetite) are of two types: amphetamines or non-amphetamines, depending on their chemical composition. Both suppress appetite by depressing the activity of certain brain areas. Both are potentially psychologically addictive; amphetamines can be chemically addictive as well.

The non-amphetamines are generally safer than the amphetamines, but both must be used with caution in the presence of epilepsy, high blood pressure, heart disease, diabetes, or pregnancy. Both types of drugs can produce insomnia, jitteriness, increased heart rate, elevated blood pressure, headaches, and nausea. Some people are unusually sensitive to the drugs, experiencing allergic reactions and sometimes even psychotic behavior. With prolonged usage, addiction may occur and serious withdrawal symptoms appear when use of the drug is discontinued.

The methyl cellulose found in most over-the-counter diet pills is not a drug and does not suppress appetite by interrupting brain patterns. Methyl cellulose is an indigestible substance which adds bulk to the diet. The idea is that this bulky material will fill the stomach and fool it into not sending out hunger pang messages.

A particularly undesirable fad has recently appeared on the diet scene — the use of thyroid hormones. These hormones stimulate metabolism causing the body to burn up calories faster than usual and, thus, sounds like a great idea for the treatment of obesity. There is, however, a hitch. In people whose thyroid functions normally, thyroid hormones produce no increase in metabolism unless given in doses which can cause serious side-effects. This therapy is, therefore, not only useless but potentially dangerous, except in those rare cases in which obesity is associated with evidence of below-normal functioning of the thyroid gland — hypothyroidism.

Diuretics have also been tried for the treatment of obesity. They will in no way affect your appetite, nor will they cause fat to disappear. The weight loss that can be seen with diuretics is strictly a result of pulling water out of the tissues. Diuretics, when used for long periods of time without medical supervision, can cause a potentially serious chemical imbalance in the body.

The use of human hormone chorionic gonadotropin, also proclaimed to "melt off the pounds," is just one more disappointment in the long quest for a weight loss miracle. You can add to this list digitalis, belladonna, and many other items pawned off on the ever hopeful obese population.

What about exercise?

Exercise plus restriction of caloric intake is the key to healthy and successful weight loss. Keep in mind, however, that if you are counting on exercise to burn up a certain number of calories, you must make the exercise a part of your daily routine. At those times when exercise is not feasible, you will need to reduce your caloric intake accordingly.

Strenuous activities such as football and swimming use up seventy-five percent more calories than activities such as studying or talking and fifty percent more calories than activities like walking or doing housework. You can use up ten calories a minute playing football or tennis or swimming, jogging, or skipping rope. Walking and playing table tennis will use up about four calories a minute. And don't think that you have to exercise for long periods at a time. Skip the elevator and walk up those stairs. A few minutes here and a few minutes there all add up. See Table 7 for more examples.

Incidentally, there is no truth to the myth that exercise will just make you hungrier. In fact, there is evidence to suggest that exercise is necessary for the accurate regulation of food intake by the appetite. Boredom is the greatest culprit in making you feel a need for physiologically unnecessary food!

Do the calories in alcohol count?

You bet they do! The addition of one beer or martini a day can add a pound of weight in three weeks.

A glass of beer contains about the same number of calories as a glass of whole milk, but without any of the milk's redeeming features of protein and calcium and other nutrients. A jigger (1½ ounces) of gin, rum, vodka, whiskey, tequila — all distilled spirits, that is — will cost you between 100 and 125 calories depending on the proof (a measure of the alcohol content) of the product. The higher the proof, the higher the calories. Three ounces of a sweet wine contain about 160 calories, whereas the same amount of dry wine contains about 85 calories.

You can cook with distilled spirits such as bourbon, plain brandy, etc., without worrying about the calories, however. Alcohol evaporates when heated, leaving little in the way of calories. Beer and wines will also give up their caloric content from the alcohol, but they leave behind their carbohydrate calories.

It's wishful thinking to believe that alcohol calories don't count. If you must drink, look for the special low-calorie (light) beers and dilute your hard liquor with water or club soda, neither of which adds additional calories. Tonic water, however, has about 80 calories per 8 ounces.

TABLE 7
CALORIC EXPENDITURE OF VARIOUS ACTIVITIES

Minimal Energy Expenditure (5 or less calories expended per minute of activity)	Moderate Energy Expenditure (5 to 10 calories expended per minute of activity)	High Energy Expenditure (more than 10 calories expended per minute of activity)
archery	basketball	football
baseball	boxing	long-distance skiing
bowling	cycling, 9.4 mph	running (jogging)
canoeing, slow	dancing	soccer
cycling, 5.5. mph	digging	skipping rope
driving	fencing	speed and endurance
gardening, light	gymnastics	cycling, 13.1 mph
general housework	high jump	speed rowing
golf	horseback riding, trot	speed skating
horseback riding, walk	riveting	squash
ironing	sawing wood	swimming
playing musical instrument	skiing	tennis, singles
sewing	stair climbing	wrestling
sitting, writing, watching TV, reading	tennis, doubles	
table tennis	walking briskly	
talking, conversation or lecturing	weight lifting	
typing		
volleyball		
walking slowly		

Seven Steps to Safe and Effective Dieting

1. *See your doctor.* There are some medical disorders which result in excess weight. It is necessary to rule out the possibility of these conditions.

The Commonsense Guide to Good Eating

Also, a weight reduction program often requires a nutritionally inadequate and unbalanced diet. Thus, before subjecting yourself to any such imbalance, it would be wise to have a thorough medical examination.

    2. *Take a long, hard look at your reasons for wanting to lose weight.* Experience has shown that overweight people with short-term goals—such as wanting to look attractive in a bathing suit for their two-week vacation, or wanting to fit into a certain outfit for a special occasion—usually do not keep the excess weight off, even though they may succeed in losing it for the special motivating event. And there is some suggestion that this yo-yoing—taking large amounts of weight off, putting it back on—may very well be more harmful to your health than consistent overweight. This is not meant to discourage you from undertaking a weight reduction program, but rather to give you a more realistic idea of what you can expect as a result of your endeavors.

    3. *Establish the caloric intake that will allow you to reduce at a safe rate.* Gaining weight is a matter of taking in more calories in food than your body needs. The body then stores these extra calories in the form of fat. To lose weight, you must take in fewer calories than your body needs so that it will draw on its stored up calories to make up the deficit—and, thus, reduce your excess fat.

    Since every pound of body fat represents about 3,500 calories, reducing your maintenance level by 500 calories a day will result in a loss of approximately one pound a week—500 calories/day x 7 days = 3,500 calories = 1 pound. Likewise, reducing your caloric intake below maintenance level by 1,000 calories will yield a loss of about two pounds a week. Table 8 may be useful.

    If you are minimally overweight, one to two pounds of weight loss per week is the maximum you should probably try for. More rapid reduction may cause your body difficulties in readjusting and you may find yourself weak and subject to easy fatigue—not to mention grouchy. (Clearly this would not be an adequate weight loss rate for the massively obese person—it would take too long to lose the weight and the person would probably abandon the effort.) Incidentally, you may well find that you lose inches before you lose pounds. So, don't be discouraged—drag out the old tape measure and rejoice!

    It is important to realize that the amount of weight lost each week will not necessarily be the same. Actually, your initial *weight* loss may be much greater than the one or two pounds a week indicated. This is due to water losses and, unfortunately, some lean muscle loss. *Fat* losses don't occur right away. Stick to your diet, however, and the fat will start to disappear. And don't be discouraged by those "plateaus" you reach occasionally wherein your weight doesn't seem to budge. Though different people lose weight at different rates even when on the identical diet, over a period of time your weight loss will average out at about the one-to-two pound a week rate.

TABLE 8
CALORIC ALLOWANCE FOR WEIGHT LOSS

Desired Weight[1]	Maintenance Calories[2]	Daily Caloric Allowance to Achieve:	
		1 lb wgt loss/wk	2 lb wgt loss/wk
100	1500	1000	500[3]
110	1650	1150	650[3]
120	1800	1300	800
130	1950	1450	950
140	2100	1600	1100
150	2250	1750	1250
160	2400	1900	1400
170	2550	2050	1550
180	2700	2200	1700
190	2850	2350	1850
200	3000	2500	2000

[1] If you use *present* weight rather than *desired* weight, you will not lose weight. You have to use up the surplus of calories you have already stored up in the form of fat.
[2] Calculated at 15 calories/pound for a minimally active person. If you are extremely inactive you may require as few as 12 calories/pound for weight maintenance.
[3] Not recommended.

---

4. *Choose a diet plan that will meet your nutritional needs if this is possible.* It is difficult to meet your nutrient supply on diets of less than 1,200 calories a day. Therefore, be especially careful about your protein intake. Also, if your caloric intake is below this level or if for some other reason it is not possible to get your vitamins and minerals through your food selection, a multi-vitamin-mineral supplement would be a good idea. Purchased by generic name (that is, not protected by a trademark) vitamin-mineral supplements are much less expensive yet equally effective as name-brand varieties. "Super" or "extra strength" formulas are not necessary or advisable unless prescribed by your doctor to treat a specific ailment.

To assist you in your food selection, foods have been grouped in the chapter on Diet Plans according to caloric and nutrient values. The foods in each group are similar enough in calories, protein, fat, and carbohydrates to be interchangeable. If you choose from these food groups the amounts indicated in the accompanying diet plans, you will be eating a nutritionally sound diet and one that will help you lose weight safely. For a thorough discussion of your nutrient needs, you may want to read the chapter on Food Selection.

5. *Establish a routine exercise pattern and stick to it!* Even a light exercise like table tennis will burn up twenty calories in five minutes. Table 7, shown earlier, lists the number of calories expended per minute for various activities.

The Commonsense Guide to Good Eating

6. *Weigh yourself regularly but not daily.* Once you have reached the weight that makes you look and feel best, continue to weigh at least weekly to make sure that you stay at that weight. This should be done in the morning after you have emptied your bladder and before you eat or drink anything. Make sure that your scales are accurate and that the adjusting knob has not been disturbed unintentionally.

Small increases in weight are sometimes the result of an unusual amount of water retained in the tissues. This occasionally happens when you have eaten very salty foods or during menstruation. This extra weight disappears in a relatively short time as the tissues release the water.

7. *Let's face it.* Occasionally you're going to blow your diet—sometimes accidentally and sometimes because you just can't stand it any more. We all go through this, and there's nothing to feel guilty about. Just cut down on your calories the next day to compensate and continue with your diet as before.

If you are consistently having trouble staying on your diet, however, try to get at the cause. Are you trying to lose weight too fast and, therefore, aren't eating enough to satisfy your appetite? Do you always overeat under the same set of circumstances—while watching TV, when bored or upset, etc.? Are you eating foods high in calories but low in satisfaction—peanuts, for example, at 100 calories for ten peanuts? Are you getting enough rest? Many people overeat when they are tired. Whatever the cause, root it out and then avoid it in the future if possible. The hints given later in this chapter may also prove helpful.

The Diet Diary

An important step in changing your eating habits is to become more aware of the food you eat, the times and places you eat, and your emotions at the time you eat. You will also probably want to set a weight-loss goal for yourself, as well as to keep a record of your progress. Keeping a diet diary can help you with these evaluations.

On page one, you should enter: the date, your height and present weight, your goal weight, the number of calories required to maintain your desired weight (see Table 6), and the number of calories required to lose weight at your desired rate (Table 8). Chest, waist, hip, thigh, and upper arm measurements should also be noted. At least once a week, weigh and remeasure yourself and enter this information in your diary.

You may also want to calculate approximately how long it will take you to reach your desired weight. This can be done by dividing the amount of weight to be lost by the number of pounds you plan to lose each week. For example: 20 pounds of excess weight $\div$ 2 pound/week loss = 10 weeks.

I'm Overweight! Now What?

A rough outline of a routine exercise plan would also be a worthwhile entry. But try to be realistic about what you're likely to really do. You'll just feel guilty and depressed when you fail to live up to unreasonable goals.

Now, divide a separate page into the following columns:

I	II	III	IV	V
Food Item	Amount Eaten	Time Eaten	Eating Place	Calories

You will want to enter in columns I and II on your paper *everything* you eat each day. This part of the diary should be kept daily for at least one week. If at any time you find that your weight is slipping back up, start this part of your diary again. Don't forget snacks, "just a taste," and nibbles. It's best if you carry your paper around with you so that you can immediately enter your food intake; otherwise, it's awfully easy to forget some of the nibbling that you do.

In columns III and IV, enter the time of day when the eating took place and where you were and/or what you were doing while eating—watching television in the living room, for example. Some people find it helpful to note how they felt while eating—mad, bored, depressed—if they are trying to identify factors that might contribute to undesirable eating habits.

At the end of each day, use the food exchange lists in the chapter on Diet Plans to find each item of food that you ate. Record on your chart the appropriate caloric "cost" of each food item. Combination foods, such as meat loaf or even french fried onions, will give you the most problem in breaking down the ingredients and amounts for inclusion in your chart. You may just have to make a "guesstimate." The easiest way to handle the problem is just to list an ounce of meat loaf as if it were an ounce of plain meat; treat the french fried onions similarly. It won't be as accurate as a breakdown of ingredients would be, but it *will be close enough for our purposes.*

Now, add up the number of calories and you are ready to compare your present eating patterns with that which will be required for you to lose weight.

Let's look first at your total daily caloric intake. How does it compare with your earlier calculation of the number of calories required for you to lose weight? Suppose your daily intake is 3,000 calories; to lose weight your intake should be only 1,500 calories. In other words, you must cut your caloric intake in half. How can you possibly do this? Let's look closely at what your food diary information reveals.

Are a lot of the items in column I what are commonly called "empty calorie" foods;—that is, foods that provide calories but little in the way of protein or vitamins and minerals? If so, can you eliminate these foods or at least substitute something lower in calories?

What about the *amount* of food eaten? Merely reducing the size of each portion can significantly reduce the total calories. Some people find the use of smaller plates helpful. Is there any correlation between the time of day and the kind and amounts of food that you eat? Do you, for example, regularly eat a candy bar after school or have a sweet roll during a mid-morning break? Maybe what you're doing or how you're feeling at the time or at the place is your problem. All of these things can provide clues as to why you eat what you eat. Use this information to your advantage!

It is also important to be realistic as to what you can expect of yourself. Many people find that they have better results if they tackle their diet program in stages. For example, a first step might be to increase your daily exercise pattern by at least fifteen minutes, without altering your food intake. A second step might be dealing with a certain problem food—such as eliminating soft drinks from your diet or at least substituting diet sodas. A third step could move you to the number of calories required for maintenance of your desired weight, while a fourth could mean going to the number of calories to reduce your weight by one pound a week. You might want then to try for a two-pound-a-week weight loss.

On the other hand, some will say that if you are committed to tackling the problem of excess fat, you should enter wholeheartedly into a weight reduction program. The decision is yours.

But what if your calculations show that you aren't taking in too many calories and yet you're clearly overweight? Then you'd better take another look at your calculations. Make sure you have made a *realistic* evaluation of your activity and growth level; check to see if your food and calorie consumption is accurate and typical of your usual eating pattern. Any way you look at it, calories in excess of body requirements lead to weight gain, while a deficit of calories will cause weight loss.

It is very common to overestimate your activity level or to forget exactly what and how much you ate in a 24-hour period. A group of overweight people who swore they were eating within their caloric allotment but not losing weight were admitted to the hospital and fed exactly what they said they had been eating. Every one of the people lost weight! They had not purposely lied or cheated, but they had miscalculated.

Hints for Changing Your Eating Habits

• Don't shop for groceries when you're hungry.
• Don't purchase "problem foods"—for example, sugar-coated cereals, candies and cookies, soft drinks. And don't be misled by foods that sound as if they are low in calories. For instance, dry-roasted peanuts, which many people

assume to be low in calories, contain approximately 172 calories in two tablespoons—only eight calories less than two tablespoons of oil-roasted peanuts at 180 calories!
- If you must have problem foods in the house for others without weight problems, don't come in contact with these foods. Let the others get their own sweets, make their own desserts, open their own soft drinks.
- Scraps or left-overs should go directly into the garbage or be stored. Don't be tempted to eat those last "few" bites—the starving children in India will not be any better off for your obesity! Leaving the table immediately after eating may prove helpful; don't hang around for a second cup of coffee.
- Make problem eating as difficult as possible. For example, if you eat bread, always toast it first—one slice at a time. And don't put serving dishes of food on the dining table. This makes second helpings too easy to come by.
- Plan your snacks, rather than eat them at random. That way, you'll feel less deprived and have something to look forward to.
- Make sure that you always have low-calorie foods on hand for when the "munchies" overcome you.
- Eat more slowly. You'll be more aware of the early signals of approaching fulness. Eat almost all foods, sandwiches included, with a fork and knife to help you eat slower. Put down your eating utensils after every bite.
- Learn to be able to refuse extra food. You can always say "it's doctor's orders."
- Don't start your weight control program on a weekend or right before a holiday. Once you're on your diet, you might want to ease up and go to your maintenance level of calories during times that you know will be difficult for you. Another approach is to eat even less immediately before the weekend or holiday feast; that way, you may be able to enjoy the meals more without feeling guilty.
- Make a "contract" with yourself—a deal wherein you reward yourself at each successful step of your diet. For example, when you've learned to eat more slowly, take an hour off to read a good book, watch the clouds roll by, or do whatever else appeals to you. Lost your first five pounds? Treat yourself to a movie or play, or spend an afternoon with your friends. You deserve a pat on the back—even if it's given by your own hand.
- Form a diet club. Get a group of your friends together who share weight control problems. It's a lot easier to map out and stick to a diet plan when you have encouragement and when you're not the only one fighting the battle of the bulge. You may find that some weight-conscious parents or teachers would like to join in this group endeavor.

As a group you may want to do nothing more than work on your diet diaries, maintain height-weight and measurement charts and help each other figure out caloric requirements and energy expenditures. There are many other possibilities, however:

1. Take turns preparing nutritious but low-calorie meals and then dine together. Your whole family will benefit from your knowledge.

2. Solicit support for a petition to your local school to post caloric values on cafeteria foods.

3. Do a study of TV food commercials and vending machine offerings to see how these influence the public's eating patterns.

4. Exercise together.

You may also want to swap tips for looking slimmer while dieting. A few hints include:

1. Women shouldn't wear very short skirts. Heavy upper legs make you look stockier than is necessary. Incidentally, bathing suits with "little boy legs" or a skirt are more becoming to heavy thighs than the more abbreviated models, regardless of how slim you may be otherwise.

2. Midriff-revealing or midriff-hugging tops should be on your list of things to avoid—they only accentuate the "positive."

3. A one-color outfit will make you look slimmer than one with a different colored top and bottom. The latter makes you look heavier because it appears to reduce your height.

4. Shoes with straps across the front make your feet look wider than they really are.

5. In general, darker clothes and hose tend to make you appear slimmer than do bright colors.

6. Avoid bold florals or plaids and horizontal stripes. Vertical stripes, however, are slimming in appearance.

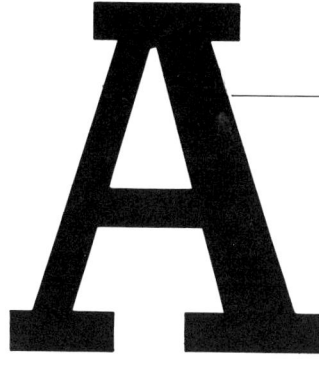# At the Store and in Your Kitchen

Practicing What We've Preached

The place at which to start putting your dietary knowledge to work is at the grocery store. Careful selection of food items, followed by thoughtful preparation will set you on the road toward a more healthful diet. The following shopping and cooking tips have been prepared by the American Heart Association. They also appear in *The American Heart Association Cookbook*,[1] a book which definitely practices what we've preached.

Shopping Tips

• Buy lean meats—fish, chicken, turkey, and veal—more often than beef, lamb, pork and ham, which contain more fat and consequently less meat per pound. Remember that you pay for that fat at the same price per pound as for the meat! Plan your menus before you shop; this saves time and cuts down on impulse buying. Take advantage of special sales. Shopping wisely can mean considerable savings.
• Restrict your use of luncheon and variety meats such as sausage, salami, frankfurters, and liverwurst, all of which have a high fat content.
• When choosing hamburger, look for the medium-to-deep color that signifies a low fat content; a light pink color is a warning that excess fat has been ground in with the meat. Or buy ground round, which is usually very lean. Better yet, select a well-trimmed piece of round steak or stewing beef, a cut that is easier on the budget, and ask the butcher to grind it for you or grind it yourself at home.
• Buy polyunsaturated vegetable oils for cooking. Safflower oil is the most polyunsaturated with soybean, corn, and cottonseed oils following in descending order. Sesame and sunflower oils are acceptable too. Where a brand name does not specify the oil, read the fine print. Some oils now on the market

are mixtures and you should know what you are buying. Olive oil is monounsaturated. It may be used in small amounts for seasoning, but it does not have the cholesterol-lowering properties of the polyunsaturates.
• Read the label before selecting a brand of margarine. The product that is high in polyunsaturates will list a recommended *liquid* vegetable oil as the first ingredient, followed by one or more partially hydrogenated vegetable oils. If the first ingredient on the list is *liquid* oil you may use the margarine. Some hydrogenation is necessary to give margarine its hardened consistency. Too much hydrogenation reduces the polyunsaturated nature of the product, transforming it into a saturated one. Tub margarines tend to be more polyunsaturated than stick margarines, since they are not required to hold a stick form. Diet margarines contain water and provide half the amount of fat found in recommended polyunsaturated margarines and consequently must be labeled *imitation*. They are usable for seasoning or as spreads but are not desirable for cooking because of their high water content.
• Read labels on packaged foods. Do not be misled by obvious ambiguity. *Vegetable fat* in a list of ingredients frequently means *saturated* vegetable fat, such as coconut oil. Be particularly careful to read the label when shopping for nondairy coffee creamers.
• Select fat-free or low-fat dairy products: skim milk, low-fat milk, evaporated skim milk, nonfat dry milk, and, despite its name, buttermilk, are all acceptable. Cheeses made from skim milk are low-fat and high in protein. These include dry cottage cheese, farmer's cheese, pot cheese, and ricotta. Parmesan cheese, mozzarella, Port du Salut, or other cheeses made from partially skimmed milk may be used in small amounts.
• Do not buy butter rolls, commercial biscuits, muffins, donuts, egg bread, cheese bread, sweet rolls, cakes, or commercial mixes containing dried eggs and whole milk.
• Convenience foods—those premixed, packaged, frozen, dehydrated, and crystallized "instant" edibles—may prove to be very inconvenient for fat-controlled eating. Read labels carefully to be certain you are not buying a product rich in saturated fat. For true convenience, no commerical product can equal nature's own fresh fruits and raw vegetables— the potato that bakes in its own jacket, the apple that needs only washing.

The following pointers will be helpful as a general shopping guide to convenience foods:

1. Any kind of packaged or prepared food that contains *no fat at all* and is otherwise allowed on your diet is all right for you to buy. Examples are vegetarian baked beans and angel food cake mix. Regular cake mixes, on the other hand, are not allowed.

2. Packaged or prepared foods *with* fat may be used only if the fat is one allowed on your diet. You may use sardines packed in cottonseed or

At the Store and in Your Kitchen

soybean oil, for example. Avoid items such as packaged popcorn, potato chips, and french fried potatoes.

3. Do not buy frozen dinners or other ready-to-eat canned or frozen food mixtures that contain fat, since you usually cannot tell what kind of fat was used, or how much.

4. Dehydrated foods, such as potatoes, and mixes to which you add the fat yourself, such as pancake mixes, are usually all right. Read the labels to be sure the product does not contain any fat.

Cooking Tips

Roasting, baking, broiling, braising, and sauteing are recommended cooking methods for meat, fish, and poultry because they require little additional fat and tend to remove interstitial fat—the fat contained in the meat.

Roasting, done in an uncovered cooking utensil in the oven, is a dry-heat method of cooking. Lean meats may require basting, but this is not usually necessary with beef, pork, or lamb, which are virtually self-basting and so lose much of their fat in a useful way during the cooking process. Always place the meat on a rack in the roasting pan to allow fat to drip away during cooking. Use low roasting temperatures (about 350°) to increase the fat drip-off. High temperatures sear the meat, sealing in the fat.

Baking, also an oven method, differs from roasting in utilizing a covered container and a little additional cooking liquid. Ideal for less fatty meats, such as lean pork chops and fish, baking retains moisture and blends flavors.

Braising and stewing are done in closed containers either in the oven or on top of the stove. More liquid is used in stewing than in braising. These are slow cooking methods excellent for tenderizing tougher cuts of meat, but they may yield unwanted fat, which stays in the cooking liquid. For this reason, it is a good idea to cook such meat dishes hours or even a day ahead of serving time, and then to refrigerate them so that hardened fat can be removed. It is less efficient to skim fat while the cooking liquid is still hot, and in many braised and stewed dishes, flavors are improved by standing.

Broiling, cooking over or under direct heat allows meat fat to drip away either into coals or into a broiling pan if a rack is used. The same result may be achieved with pan-broiling if the pan has a ridged surface. Less tender meats may be broiled after being cubed, scored, pounded, ground, or marinated. Fruit juices or wine make excellent marinades.

Saute, from the French *sauter* meaning "to jump" refers to a pan method using so little fat that food is constantly agitated or made to jump in the pan to prevent sticking. Chinese stir-frying has the same objective — to keep the food in motion so that it will not burn.

Frying is usually avoided in low-fat cookery. This is because it often involves the use of batters that can absorb the cooking fat. Instead, foods to be fried or deep-fried may be dredged in flour, or dipped in egg white and then in cracker meal. Corn oil is a good choice for deep-fat frying because its smoking point is higher than the correct cooking temperature for most foods. Fat that begins to smoke releases undesirable chemicals and will not cook correctly. When cooked until done and not overdone, food absorbs only a minimal amount of oil. It will absorb excessive amounts only if it is immersed too long or if the oil is improperly heated. The food itself will lower the fat temperature. Use a thermometer so that you will know when the correct frying temperature has been reached and allow it to return to that correct temperature before adding each new batch of food. Timing is important. Watch carefully for the moment of doneness.

Meat drippings can be useful. The rich meat essence that drips into the roasting pan or broiler along with the fat from roasts, steaks, or other meats, may be salvaged for future use by pouring the contents of the pan, fat and all, into a refrigerator dish and chilling it. The dark, protein-rich juice that separates out beneath the fat will add zest to meat pies, brown sauces, hashes or meat loaves, and soup and will be a help in using leftover meats. Discard the hardened fat.

Gravies: it is possible to make a thickened gravy without that seemingly indispensable meat fat to blend with the thickening agent. Use a cup or so of clear defatted broth — canned, made from bouillon cubes or, best of all, homemade. In a jar with a tight fitting lid place 1 tablespoon of cornstarch, or 1 tablespoon of uncooked flour, or 1 to 2 tablespoons of browned flour for each ½ cup of liquid. Shake until smooth. Heat the remaining liquid in a saucepan, pour flour mixture into it and simmer, adding seasonings as desired. Flour is browned to give the sauce a mahogany color where desired. This can be done by placing flour in a shallow pan over low heat, stirring frequently, or in an oven at 300° for about 15 minutes.

Broth: rich, homemade broth is heartier and more flavorful than the canned variety. Make it the day before you plan to use it to allow for defatting after refrigeration. Use it to make soups or stews, defatting the finished dish whenever necessary. Canned broth as well as canned soups and stews are usually relatively free of fat, but to be sure, refrigerate the can before opening it, then remove any visible fat before using the product.

Trim all visible fat from meats before cooking. Much fat will remain as interstitial marbling although it may not be obvious to the eye, and this will lubricate the meat sufficiently during cooking.

Other Cooking Hints

Wines and spirits for cooking: The wines and spirits you cook with need not be very old or expensive but they should be good enough for you to drink and enjoy.

Vinegar: Try a good wine or herb vinegar for salads.

Whole-grain flour should be kept in the refrigerator or in the freezer to keep it from becoming rancid. You may substitute 1 cup of whole wheat *pastry flour* for 1 cup all-purpose flour. You may substitute 1 cup whole wheat flour for $\frac{7}{8}$ cup all-purpose flour.

Iodized salt should be used to add this essential nutrient to your diet. Put a few grains of rice in the salt shaker to keep it free flowing.

Beans: Soak dried beans in water overnight; they'll cook in less time the next day.

Syrup: Save the juice off canned fruit; keep it frozen until needed. When ready to make your own syrup for pancakes or French toast, simply thaw the liquid, thicken it with a bit of cornstarch, and serve hot. (It's good over cooked carrots, too).

Celery: Don't throw the leaves away. Dehydrate chopped leaves in your oven at low heat. Store dried leaves until needed for soups or salads.

Vegetables: The less water used and the shorter the cooking period, the less flavor and nutrients lost. Try steaming your vegetables instead of boiling them.

Spiced fruits: Keep in the refrigerator a jar of dried fruit soaked in wine and spiced to your taste. It will come in handy to dress up rice or other foods.

Low-fat white sauce: Blend flour with a small amount of cold skim milk. Stir into remaining milk. Cook until thickened, stirring often.

Low-fat vegetables: Substitute lemon juice and/or crushed herbs for butter or margarine to flavor vegetables.

Stir-fried vegetables: Try cooking vegetables the Oriental way. Thinly slice or break vegetables into small pieces (let your imagination run wild when choosing the vegetables); then quickly cook in a small amount of oil until the vegetables are tender crisp.

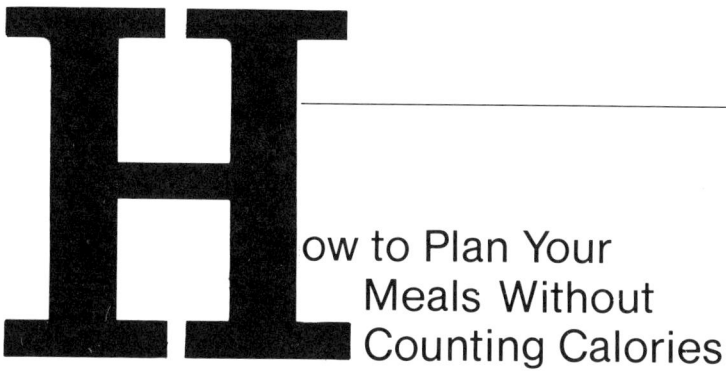

How to Plan Your Meals Without Counting Calories

Food Exchange System

The food exchange system was originally developed in 1950 to make easier the job of calculating diets for diabetics. Since that time, this method has been used by many in weight control programs. It is also a very appropriate system to use for those striving for a more balanced and acceptable diet.

The food exchange system is based on the concept of grouping together foods that are similar in calories, protein, fats, and carbohydrates. Foods within each group can, thus, be interchanged or exchanged to allow for individual preferences. For example, in the Bread Group, ½ bagel equals "1 bread exchange," as does ½ cup grits, ½ cup spaghetti, or 1 cup popcorn. Each bread exchange contains approximately 68 calories, 2 grams protein, negligible fats, and 15 grams carbohydrates.

Let's look at another example. What do 1 hot dog, 1 ounce of cheddar cheese, 1 egg, ¼ cup tuna, and 2 tablespoons of peanut butter have in common? Each contains approximately 73 calories, 7 grams protein, 5 grams fat, and almost no carbohydrates. Each equals "1 meat exchange."

There are seven exchange lists: Milk, Vegetables, Fruit, Bread, Meat, Fat, and Free Foods. After consulting the diet plans later in this chapter, you will know how many of each type of food exchange you are allowed each day. Most people find that keeping up with the number of food exchanges is much easier than counting calories and grams of protein or worrying about vitamin and mineral intakes. Once you've used the system for a while, you'll be surprised at how easy it is to remember. You'll even be able to figure out how to account for foods that aren't on the lists. So, let's jump right in and look at the exchange lists. You may want to tape copies of these lists up in your kitchen for ready reference.

List 1: Milk Exchanges

Foods in this group are high in protein, carbohydrates, and fats—unless made

The Commonsense Guide to Good Eating

from skimmed or low-fat milk. Milk will not only help supply you with protein, but will help protect your supply of calcium, phosphorus, magnesium, vitamins A, D, B^{12}, and riboflavin.

Approximate composition of 1 exchange: 170 calories for whole milk products, 80-125 calories for skim or low-fat products, 8 grams protein, 10 grams fat*, 12 grams carbohydrates

MILK		MILK, EVAPORATED	
whole	1 cup	whole	½ cup
low-fat (2%)*	1 cup	skim*	½ cup
skim (non-fat)*	1 cup	BUTTERMILK	
soybean	1 cup	whole	1 cup
MILK, POWDERED		skim*	1 cup
whole	¼ cup	YOGHURT, PLAIN	
skim*	¼ cup	whole	1 cup
soybean	¼ cup	low-fat*	1 cup

*Products made from skim milk contain almost no fat, and thus, are called for in the following diet plans to help control the amount of saturated fat and cholesterol in your diet. If you desire to use whole milk products instead, you will need to omit 2 fat exchanges from your diet plan. When using low-fat milk products, you will only need to omit 1 fat exchange.

List 2: Vegetable Exchanges

The vegetables have been divided into three groups. Group A vegetables contain little carbohydrates, protein, fat, or calories, but are important sources of vitamins and minerals. Group B vegetables, also a source of vitamins and minerals, contain a small amount of protein, moderate carbohydrates, negligible fats, and about 36 calories per half-cup. The third group of vegetables are included in List 4, Bread Exchanges, because their values are similar to bread.

Group A vegetables

When eaten raw, Group A vegetables can be eaten without worrying about amounts. If cooked, you may eat 1 cup without counting calories. Each additional cup should be counted as 1 Group B exchange.

Alfalfa sprouts
Asparagus
Bamboo shoots
Bean sprouts
Broccoli*+

Brussel sprouts
Cabbage
Cauliflower
Celery
Chicory*

How to Plan Your Meals Without Counting Calories

Chives	Mushrooms	
Cucumbers	Okra	
Eggplant	Parsley	
Endive	Peppers*+	
Escarole*	Pimento	
Fennel	Radishes	
Greens	Rhubarb	
beet greens	Romaine	
chard, Swiss	Sauerkraut	
collards+	Squash, summer	
dandelion	Squash, zucchini	
kale+	String beans	
mustard	Tomatoes	
poke	Tomato juice	½ cup
spinach	Water chestnuts	3
turnip greens+	Watercress*	
Kohlrabi	Wax beans	
Lettuce		

Group B vegetables

One-half cup, raw or cooked, equals 1 exchange except where noted otherwise. One Group B vegetable exchange can be substituted for one-half of a Bread exchange.

Approximate composition of 1 exchange: 36 calories, 2 grams protein, 0 grams fat, 7 grams carbohydrates

Artichokes	1 whole	Snowpeas	
Beets		Soybeans	
Carrots*		Squash, winter	
Miso (fermented rice & soybeans)	1 tbsp.	Squash, acorn, butternut, hubbard	
		Tomato catsup	1½ tbsp.
Onions		Tomato paste	3 tbsp.
Peas, green		Tomato sauce	
Pumpkin*		Turnips	
Rutabagas		V-8 juice	⅔ cup

List 3: Fruit Exchanges

Approximate composition of 1 exchange: 40 calories, 0 grams protein, 0 grams fat, 10 grams carbohydrates. One fruit exchange may be substituted for ⅔ bread exchange.

*High vitamin A content. Should have at least one serving every other day.
+High vitamin C content.

The Commonsense Guide to Good Eating

APPLE		peach nectar	½ cup
fresh	1 sm.	pear nectar	⅓ cup
sauce	½ cup	pineapple	⅓ cup
APRICOTS		prune	¼ cup
canned	½ cup	tangerine	½ cup
dried	4 halves	tomato	½ cup
fresh	3 sm.	*LYCHEE FRUIT*	4
BANANA	½ sm.	*MANGO+*	½ sm.
BERRIES		*MELON*	
blackberries	1 cup	cantaloupe+	½ sm.
blueberries	⅔ cup	honeydew+	¼ med.
boysenberries	1 cup	watermelon	1 cup diced
cranberries	1 cup	*NECTARINE*	1 med.
gooseberries	1 cup	*ORANGES*	
loganberries	1 cup	fresh, whole+	1 med.
raspberries	1 cup	mandarin, canned	¾ cup
strawberries+	1 cup	sections, fresh or	
CHERRIES		canned+	½ cup
sour	½ cup	*PAPAYA*	1/3 med.
sweet	10 large	*PEACHES*	
CRANBERRY SAUCE	2 tbsp.	canned	½ cup
DATES	2	dried	2 halves
FIGS		fresh, whole	1 med.
canned	½ cup	fresh, sliced	½ cup
dried	1 sm.	*PERSIMMON*	½ med.
fresh	2 lg.	*PINEAPPLE*	
FRUIT COCKTAIL	½ cup	canned	½ cup or 1 slice
GRAPES		fresh	½ cup or 1 slice
canned	⅓ cup	*PLUMS*	
fresh	15 or ½ cup	canned	½ cup
GRAPEFRUIT+	½ med.	fresh	2 med.
GUAVA	⅔	*POMEGRANATE*	1 sm.
JUICES		*PRUNES*	2 med.
apple	½ cup	*RAISINS*	2 tbsp.
apricot nectar	⅓ cup	*TANGERINES*	
grape	¼ cup	fresh, whole	2 sm.
grapefruit+	½ cup	sections	½ cup
orange+	½ cup		

+Rich source of vitamin C.

How to Plan Your Meals Without Counting Calories

List 4: Bread Exchanges

This list includes high carbohydrate foods such as breads, cereals, spaghetti, crackers, dried beans and peas, and some other vegetables. One bread exchange may be substituted for 2 group B vegetable exchanges *or* 1½ fruit exchanges.

Approximate composition of 1 exchange: 68 calories, 2 grams protein, 0 grams fat, 15 grams carbohydrates

BREADS, ROLLS, ETC.
bagel	½
banana bread[1]	1 slice
biscuit	1
bread: white, rye, pumpernickel, whole wheat	1 slice
bread: Italian, French, Vienna	1½ slices
bread sticks (9" long)	4
challa	1 slice
cornbread	1½ in. cube
English muffin	½
hamburger roll	½
hotdog roll	½
muffin	1
popover	1
raisin bread, no icing	1 slice
spoonbread	½ cup
tortilla	1

CEREALS
cooked	½ cup
dry, flake	⅔ cup
dry, puffed	1½ cups
shredded wheat	1 lg. biscuit
wheat germ	2 tbsp.

CRACKERS, COOKIES
animal	8
ginger snaps	2
graham	1
matzos (6 in.)	1
melba toast	4
oatmeal cookies[1]	2
oyster	20
peanut butter cookies[1]	2
pretzels	10 very thin or 1 lg.
round, thin	6
rye, whole grain	3
saltines	5
soda	3
sugar cookies	2
vanilla wafers	5

DESSERTS
brownie, no icing[2]	1
flavored gelatin	½ cup
ice cream[2]	½ cup
ice cream cone, wafer	2
ice milk[1]	½ cup
poundcake, no icing[1]	1 slice
sherbert	¼ cup
sponge or angel food cake	1½ in. cube

FLOUR PRODUCTS
Bisquick	¾ oz.
corn meal	3 tbsp.
cornstarch	2 tbsp.
flour, all-purpose	2½ tbsp.
Matzo meal	3 tbsp.
rye flour	4 tbsp.
tapioca, dry	2 tbsp.

PASTA, RICE, ETC.
barley, cooked	½ cup
cracked wheat (bulgur), dry	2 tbsp.
Kasha, cooked	½ cup
macaroni, cooked	½ cup
rice, cooked	½ cup

[1]Omit 1 fat exchange from daily diet allowance.
[2]Omit 2 fat exchanges from daily diet allowance.

The Commonsense Guide to Good Eating

spaghetti, cooked	½ cup	potatoes, french fried	10

SOUP
canned, undiluted	½ cup		

MISCELLANEOUS
bread stuffing[1]	½ cup
carob powder	4 tbsp.
corn, popped, without butter	1 cup
doughnut, plain[1]	1
enchilada	1
french toast[1]	1 slice
pancake (3" diam.)	2
pizza, plain[1]	⅙ pie
potato chips[2]	1 oz. (15 chips)
tacos	1
tamale	1
waffle	1

VEGETABLES
baked beans, no pork	¼ cup
beans, peas, lentils, dried, cooked	½ cup
beans, lima, fresh, cooked	½ cup
corn, sweet	⅓ cup or ½ ear
mixed vegetables	½ cup
parsnips	⅔ cup
potato, white	1 whole or ½ cup mashed
potato, sweet or yam	½ whole or ¼ cup mashed

[1]Omit 1 fat exchange from daily diet allowance.
[2]Omit 2 fat exchanges from daily diet allowance.

List 5: Meat Exchanges

This list includes a variety of foods, moderately high in protein and fat content. The quantities refer to ready-to-eat weight. Bones and extra fat are not counted in the serving weight. To allow for shrinkage, figure that about 4 or 5 ounces of most raw meats will provide 3 ounces of cooked meat.

> Approximate composition of 1 exchange: 73 calories, 7 grams protein, 5 grams fat*, 0 grams carbohydrate

*MEAT AND POULTRY, COOKED***
beef, ham, lamb, pork, veal, fowl, liver, etc.	1 oz.
beef, dried, chipped[1]	2 thin slices
canadian bacon	1 slice
cold cuts	1 slice ⅛" thick
corned beef, pastrami	1 oz.
hot dog (8-9/lb)	1
meat ball	1 sm.
sausage, pork[2]	2 sm. links
deviled ham, canned	2 rounded tbsp.

EGG   1 (4 egg whites)

SEAFOOD
clams, oysters, shrimp	5
cod, haddock, halibut, herring, gelfiltefish, flounder, catfish	1 oz.

[1]Low in fat content. You may add 1 fat exchange to your daily diet.
[2]High in fat content. Omit 2 fat exchanges from your daily diet.
*Remember that fatty meats, organ meats, cold cuts, hot dogs, sausage, poultry skin, crab, shrimp, lobster, egg yolks, and whole milk cheeses are high in saturated fat and cholesterol.
**One-half large breast of chicken equals approximately 3 ounces. One thigh plus one drumstick equals approximately 3 ounces. A standard serving of meat is usually about 3 ounces.

How to Plan Your Meals Without Counting Calories

crab, lobster, salmon, tuna, dried squid	¼ cup	soy cheese (tofu)	¼ cup
frog legs	2 lg.	PEANUT BUTTER	2 tbsp.
herring, pickled	1¼ oz.	PEANUTS	20
sardines	3	SOYBEANS, dried (1¼ cup, cooked).	½ cup
CHEESE			
american, cheddar, swiss	1 oz., 1 slice, 1″ cube, or ¼ cup grated	VEGEBURGER	2 tbsp.
cheese spreads	2 tbsp.	BREWER'S YEAST	3 tbsp.
cottage cheese	¼ cup		

List 6: Fat Exchanges

Approximate composition of 1 exchange: 45 calories, 0 grams protein, 5 grams fat*, 0 grams carbohydrate

AVOCADO	⅛	OILS AND COOKING FATS	1 tsp.
BACON, CRISP	1 slice	OLIVES	
BUTTER OR MARGARINE		green	10 med.
regular	1 tsp.	black	6 med.
diet type	2 tsp.	PIGS FEET	1
CHOCOLATE, BITTER**	⅓ ounce	SALAD DRESSINGS	
COCONUT, FRESH	1″ cube	french, italian, regular	1 tbsp.
CREAM		french, italian, low-calorie type	4 tbsp.
half and half	2 tbsp.	rouquefort (blue cheese), regular	2 tsp.
sour	2 tbsp.	rouquefort, low-calorie type	4 tbsp.
whipped	1 tbsp.	thousand island, regular	2 tsp.
CREAM CHEESE		thousand island, low-calorie type	2 tbsp.
regular	1 tbsp.		
low-calorie type	2 tbsp.		
DIPS, READY-TO-SERVE	2 tbsp	SALT PORK	¾ in. cube
GRAVIES AND SAUCES	2 tbsp.	SEEDS	
MAYONNAISE		pumpkin	1½ tbsp.
regular	1 tsp.	sesame	1 tbsp.
low-calorie type	2 tbsp.	sunflower	1½ tbsp.
NUTS***	6 sm.	TARTAR SAUCE	1½ tsp.

*Remember that animal fats, products containing egg yolks or whole milk, chocolate, coconut, and coconut and palm oils are all high in saturated fat and cholesterol.
**See "carob powder" in List 4: Bread Exchanges. It is an excellent substitute for chocolate — lower in calories and fat.
***Peanuts are a source of protein and will be found in List 5: Meat Exchanges.

List 7: Free Foods

The foods in this list contain only negligible amounts of calories, protein, carbohydrates, and fat and may be used as desired.

Bouillon and broth, fat free[1]
Coffee
Diet jellies
Dill pickles
Gelatin, low-calorie or unflavored
Group A vegetables, raw
Herbs and spices
Horseradish

Lemon
Mustard
Non-caloric sweeteners
Soy sauce[1]
Sugar-free soft drinks
Sugarless chewing gum
Tea
Vinegar

[1]High in salt content.

Miscellaneous Exchanges

The foodstuffs in this list are primarily sources of concentrated carbohydrates, providing calories but little else of nutrient value. *Diabetics should consult their physicians before using any of these products and before adopting any diet plan.*

    Alcoholic beverages can really eat into your calorie allowance. For example, look at the following:

ALCOHOLIC BEVERAGES[1]
ale	8 oz. = 1½
beer	8 oz. = 1½
brandy	1 oz. = 1½
cordials	1 oz. = 1½
liquor: gin, rum, scotch, vodka, whiskey	1½ oz. = 1½
manhattan	3½ oz. = 2
martini	3½ oz. = 2
vermouth	3½ oz. = 2

WINES
port, muscatelle	3½ oz. = 1
sauterne, champagne, claret, chablis	3½ oz. = 1
sherry	2 oz. = 1

*HONEY, MOLASSES**[1]   1½ tbsp. = 1

JAMS AND JELLIES[2]   1 tbsp. = 1

REGULAR COLA DRINKS[1]   6 oz. = 1

SUGAR[1]   3½ tsp. = 1

*Blackstrap molasses is, however, a good source of calcium, iron, and the B vitamins.
[1]The equivalents are shown in terms of bread exchanges.
[2]The equivalent is shown in terms of a fruit exchange.

How to Plan Your Meals Without Counting Calories

You can easily fit your favorite foods into the Exchange Lists. Nutritional composition information on food labels or other food composition tables will allow you to place the food in the appropriate list according to calorie, protein, carbohydrate, and fat content. And don't worry about the food not having the exact nutritional composition as that shown for a particular list. These values are only averages—the food items within each list vary, so you have a certain amount of leeway for "guesstimating." Also, many manufacturers will supply you with a list of their products showing how they can be fitted into the Exchange Lists.

One especially complete source of food composition tables is: Church, C.F. and Church, H.N. *Food Values of Portions Commonly Used*. Philadelphia: J.B. Lippincott Company, 1970.

The United States Department of Agriculture also puts out a book of food values: *Nutritive Value of Foods*. Home and Garden Bulletin No. 72, 1971, available for sale (75¢) by the Superintendent of Documents, US Government Printing Office, Washington, D.C. 20402.

Diet Plans Tailored to Your Individual Food Preferences

In keeping with our present knowledge about the relationship of nutrition to health, each of the following diet plans provides at least 50 grams of protein—in fact, all but the 800 and 1000 calorie diets contain at least 70 grams of protein—and no more than 35% of the calories come from fats. Carbohydrates range between 39 and 44% of the total calories. Additionally, the sample menus have been designed to minimize the amounts of saturated fats and cholesterol. Where a diet plan is known to be deficient in certain nutrients, a note to this effect is included.

DIET PLANS

Exchange List	Number of Exchanges	Calories	Composition of Exchanges		
			Protein gm	Fat gm	Carb. gm
800-Calorie Diet					
Milk[1]	☐ ☐	176	16	–	24
Vegetable B[2]	☐	36	2	–	7
Fruit	☐ ☐	80	–	–	20
Bread	☐ ☐	136	4	–	30
Meat	☐ ☐ ☐ ☐ ☐	365	35	25	–
Fat	None	–	–	–	–
		793	57	25	81
			29%	28%	41%

83

The Commonsense Guide to Good Eating

Exchange List	Number of Exchanges	Calories	Composition of Exchanges		
			Protein gm	Fat gm	Carb. gm

1000-Calorie Diet

Exchange List	Number of Exchanges	Calories	Protein gm	Fat gm	Carb. gm
Milk[1]	☐ ☐	176	16	-	24
Vegetable B[2]	☐	36	2	-	7
Fruit	☐ ☐	80	-	-	20
Bread	☐ ☐ ☐	204	6	-	45
Meat	☐ ☐ ☐ ☐ ☐	438	42	30	-
Fat	☐	45	-	5	-
		979	66	35	96
			27%	32%	39%

1200-Calorie Diet

Exchange List	Number of Exchanges	Calories	Protein gm	Fat gm	Carb. gm
Milk[1]	☐ ☐	176	16	-	24
Vegetable B[2]	☐ ☐	72	4	-	14
Fruit	☐ ☐ ☐	120	-	-	30
Bread	☐ ☐ ☐ ☐	272	8	-	60
Meat	☐ ☐ ☐ ☐ ☐	438	42	30	-
Fat	☐ ☐	90	-	10	-
		1168	70	40	128
			24%	31%	44%

1500-Calorie Diet

Exchange List	Number of Exchanges	Calories	Protein gm	Fat gm	Carb. gm
Milk[1]	☐ ☐ + ¼	198	18	-	27
Vegetable B[2]	☐ ☐	72	4	-	14
Fruit	☐ ☐ ☐	120	-	-	30
Bread	☐ ☐ ☐ ☐ ☐	408	12	-	90
Meat	☐ ☐ ☐ ☐ ☐ ☐	511	49	35	-
Fat	☐ ☐ ☐ ☐	180	-	20	-
		1489	83	55	161
			22%	33%	43%

[1] Skimmed milk is called for in all diet plans except for those trying to gain weight. Not only will this save on calories, but it will also help reduce the amount of saturated fat and cholesterol in your diet. If you wish to use whole milk instead, you will need to omit 2 fat exchanges from your diet plan. Low-fat products call for the omission of 1 fat exchange.

[2] Group A vegetables can be eaten freely as long as they are raw. When cooked, 2 cups of Group A vegetables are equal to 1 Group B vegetable exchange.

How to Plan Your Meals Without Counting Calories

Exchange List	Number of Exchanges	Composition of Exchanges			
		Calories	Protein gm	Fat gm	Carb. gm
2000-Calorie Diet					
Milk[1]	☐☐☐	264	24	-	36
Vegetable B[2]	☐☐	72	4	-	14
Fruit	☐☐☐	120	-	-	30
Bread	☐☐☐☐☐☐☐☐	612	18	-	135
Meat	☐☐☐☐☐☐☐☐	657	63	45	-
Fat	☐☐☐☐☐	270	-	30	-
		1995	109	75	215
			22%	34%	43%
2500-Calorie Diet					
Milk[1]	☐☐☐	264	24	-	36
Vegetable B[2]	☐☐☐	108	6	-	21
Fruit	☐☐☐	120	-	-	30
Bread	☐☐☐☐☐☐☐☐☐☐☐☐	816	24	-	180
Meat	☐☐☐☐☐☐☐☐☐☐☐	876	84	60	-
Fat	☐☐☐☐☐☐☐	315	-	35	-
		2499	138	95	267
			22%	34%	43%
3000-Calorie Diet					
Milk[1]	☐☐☐☐	352	32	-	48
Vegetable B[2]	☐☐☐	108	6	-	21
Fruit	☐☐☐☐	160	-	-	40
Bread	☐☐☐☐☐☐☐☐☐☐☐☐☐☐	952	28	-	210
Meat	☐☐☐☐☐☐☐☐☐☐☐☐☐☐	1022	98	70	-
Fat	☐☐☐☐☐☐☐☐☐	405	-	45	-
		2999	164	115	319
			22%	35%	43%

[1] Skimmed milk is called for in all diet plans except for those trying to gain weight. Not only will this save on calories, but it will also help reduce the amount of saturated fat and cholesterol in your diet. If you wish to use whole milk instead, you will need to omit 2 fat exchanges from your diet plan. Low-fat products call for the omission of 1 fat exchange.

[2] Group A vegetables can be eaten freely as long as they are raw. When cooked, 2 cups of Group A vegetables are equal to 1 Group B vegetable exchange.

The Commonsense Guide to Good Eating

For those who are trying to lose weight, we have found that it helps if you make up — on small pieces of paper that will fit in your purse, wallet, or pocket — daily diet and exercise plans. Just check off the appropriate box as you eat and exercise during the day.

The following gives cycling (a stationary bicycle is a real help if your budget will allow it) and table tennis as examples of exercise. When you make up your own plans, substitute whatever form of exercise that appeals most to you and that you're likely to perform. Table 7 (page 61), may prove helpful.

At the end of each day, you will know whether or not you have stayed on your diet. This day-by-day analysis may help you keep your diet on track.

1200-CALORIE DIET

Food		Exercise[1]	
Milk	☐ ☐	cycling, 5 mi/hr.	☐ ☐ ☐ ☐ ☐
Veg. B	☐ ☐	table tennis	☐ ☐ ☐ ☐ ☐
Fruit	☐ ☐ ☐		
Bread	☐ ☐ ☐ ☐		
Meat	☐ ☐ ☐ ☐ ☐		
Fat	☐ ☐		

[1]Each box is the equivalent of 5 minutes of exercise, or a bonus of 20 calories burned up.

Sample Menus

The following sample menus for an 800- and a 1000-calorie diet are included to give you an idea of how your choices of foods from the various exchange lists can be combined to make interesting and tasty meals. The recipes in the Appendix will also serve as further examples of the identification of nutritional composition through the use of the food exchange system. As use of the food exchange concept spreads, more and more cookbooks are starting to appear with recipes that are broken down into food exchanges. One especially nice book is: Jones, J. *The Calculating Cook.* San Francisco: 101 Productions, 1972.

800-Calorie Diet

This extremely low-calorie diet is low in iron, thiamine, and riboflavin and borderline in other nutrients. If this diet is to be followed for any length of time, a vitamin-mineral supplement should be taken daily.

How to Plan Your Meals Without Counting Calories

COMPOSITION OF 800-CALORIE DIET

This Diet Provides Approximately		Total Food Allowance for One Day	
		Exchange List	No. of Exchanges
Protein	57 grams	Milk	☐ ☐
Fat	25 grams	Grp. A Vegetables	as desired
Carbohydrates	81 grams	Grp. B Vegetables	☐
		Fruit	☐ ☐
		Bread	☐ ☐
		Meat	☐ ☐ ☐ ☐ ☐
		Fat	not allowed
		Free Foods	as desired

SAMPLE DISTRIBUTION OF FOOD EXCHANGES OVER DAY

Meal	Milk	Veg. A	Veg. B	Fruit	Bread	Meat	Fat	Free Foods
BREAKFAST Milkshake made by blending: 1 cup skim milk 1 cup strawberries artificial sweetner if desired	1			1				x
LUNCH Bouillon ½ english muffin, topped with: mustard ¼ cup tuna 1 slice cheese · heat until cheese melts Sliced tomatoes Non-caloric drink of choice		x			1	1 1		x x x
AFTERNOON SNACK 1 apple, cored and filled with 2 tbsp. peanut butter				1			1	
DINNER Skillet casserole made of: 2 oz. cooked and crumbled lean ground beef 1 cup french style string beans			x			2		

87

The Commonsense Guide to Good Eating

Meal	Milk	Veg. A	Veg. B	Fruit	Bread	Meat	Fat	Free Foods
mushrooms		x						
bean sprouts		x						
seasoned with herbs and spices to taste							x	
½ cup cooked or raw carrots			1					
Salad made of raw cauliflower		x						
Flavored with lemon juice, salt and pepper							x	
EVENING SNACK*								
5 vanilla wafers					1			
1 cup milk	1							
TOTAL "EXCHANGES"	2	x	1	2	2	5	0	x

*Some studies suggest that food eaten late in the day may turn to fat, whereas food eaten earlier in the day is efficiently utilized. You may, therefore, want to consider omitting a bedtime snack or to eat the snack food earlier in the day.

1000-Calorie Diet

This low-calorie diet is low in iron, thiamine, and riboflavin and borderline in other nutrients. If this diet is to be followed for any length of time, a vitamin-mineral supplement should be taken daily.

COMPOSITION OF 1000-CALORIE DIET

This Diet Provides Approximately		Total Food Allowance for One Day	
		Exchange List	No. of Exchanges
Protein	66 grams	Milk	☐ ☐
Fat	35 grams	Grp. A Vegetables	as desired
Carbohydrates	96 grams	Grp. B Vegetables	☐
		Fruit	☐ ☐
		Bread	☐ ☐ ☐
		Meat	☐ ☐ ☐ ☐ ☐
		Fat	☐
		Free Foods	as desired

How to Plan Your Meals Without Counting Calories

SAMPLE DISTRIBUTION OF FOOD EXCHANGES OVER DAY

Meal	Milk	Veg. A	Veg. B	Fruit	Bread	Meat	Fat	Free Foods
BREAKFAST ½ cup of prepared grits, topped with: 1 egg** and 1 tsp. diet margarine (bake at 350 for about 15-20 mins.) ½ cup orange juice				1	1	1	½	
LUNCH 2 slices dried beef, wrapped around 1 oz. low-fat cheese, and then wrapped with 1 refrigerator "crescent" roll and then baked 1 cup skim milk	1				1	1 1		
AFTERNOON SNACK 1 slice raisin bread 1 cup skim milk	1				1			
DINNER 3 oz. cooked chicken 1 broiled tomato seasoned with soy sauce 1 cooked artichoke, served with 2 tbsp. low-calorie Italian dressing Non-caloric drink of choice		x	1			3	½	x x
*EVENING SNACK** ½ grapefruit, artifically sweetened if desired				1				x
TOTAL "EXCHANGES"	2	x	1	2	3	6	1	x

*Some studies suggest that food eaten late in the day may turn to fat, whereas food eaten earlier in the day is efficiently utilized. You may, therefore, want to consider omitting a bedtime snack or to eat the snack food earlier in the day.
**Try not to exceed three eggs per week.

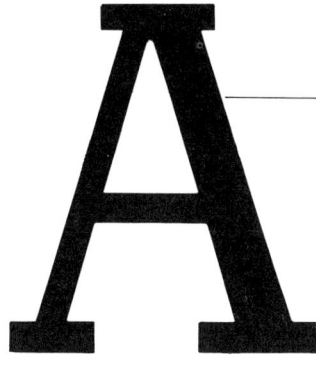# Atherosclerosis—Prevention Begins at an Early Age

A Disease That Probably Begins in Childhood

Atherosclerosis is a disease of the arteries, a condition in which fat accumulates in the wall of the artery, producing thickening, narrowing, and loss of elasticity. When this happens, the artery may gradually close altogether or a blood clot may form in the narrowed vessel, shutting off the supply of blood with its oxygen and nutrients to the part of the body served by the blood vessel. If this occurs in the arteries supplying the brain, senility or a stroke may result. If the site is in the lower extremities, gangrene can occur.

If a clot is formed in one of the small coronary arteries that nourish the heart muscle, a portion of the heart muscle will die. If the damage is extensive, the heart may be unable to function and the person dies. If the damage is small or if the person has a well-developed circulatory system due to regular strenuous exercise, the heart may be able to continue to pump blood and the muscle will heal. Thus, some people survive "myocardial infarctions" or "heart attacks" while for other people they prove fatal.

Heart disease continues to be the leading cause of death in the United States. There are a number of different kinds of heart disease associated with atherosclerosis. And there is increasing evidence to suggest that atherosclerosis begins in childhood. For example, autopsies done on very young children who died from accidents, etc., show the beginnings of some of the disease processes that might have claimed their lives in later years had they survived infancy. Also, autopsies done on soldiers in their 20s, who died of war injuries, revealed a large amount of coronary atherosclerosis. Hence, the importance of understanding better the known causes and preventions of this process.

Factors Involved

Many risk factors are involved in the incidence of atherosclerosis, heart disease, and heart attacks seen in this country: genetic factors, high blood cholesterol and triglyceride levels, elevated blood pressure, lack of exercise, obesity, excessive intake of saturated fats, tension, smoking, and diabetes. Luckily, we have a fair degree of control over many of these factors. Let's look at each one.

Family history

An important "marker" of individuals at increased risk of development of atherosclerosis is their genetic heritage. At one extreme, an individual may have had both parents who died at a relatively young age from heart attacks due to atherosclerosis of the arteries of the heart. The likelihood of this individual developing atherosclerosis is very high, especially for women whose mothers had myocardial infarctions before menopause. At the other extreme is the individual who is fortunate enough to have parents who lived to a ripe old age without any evidence of heart disease or strokes. The outlook for this individual is very good and the probability of developing atherosclerosis at an early age is less than average.

In addition to genetic factors that may contribute to atherosclerosis, family sharing of environmental risk factors—a poor diet, for example—should be looked at when any disease strikes a number of family members. No doubt even inherited susceptibility is often complicated by dietary abuses, as well as other life-style factors. We can't do anything about hereditary influence per se, but we can make other adjustments so as not to add to the problem.

Incidentally, in families susceptible to heart disease, there is often a high incidence of hypertension (high blood pressure) and diabetes. If you have a strong family history of such problems, you would be especially wise to take a look at your eating, exercise, and smoking habits.

Cholesterol levels

Cholesterol is a normal fatlike substance found in animal fats such as the fat in meat, eggs, cheese, butter, cream, and whole milk. Liver, brains, kidneys and shellfish also contain cholesterol. The most concentrated source, however, is egg yolks. Cholesterol is also manufactured by the body. A person's blood cholesterol level is, therefore, dependent on cholesterol from within (endogenous—made by their own body) and cholesterol from without (exogenous—from food sources).

If your diet contains a large amount of saturated fat (see Chapter 2 for how to identify different kinds of fat), your cholesterol level will go up. If you decrease the amount of saturated fat in your diet, your cholesterol level will go down, at least for a time. Polyunsaturated fats will help to reduce newly formed cholesterol. Other factors affecting cholesterol levels are: heredity, certain disease processes, female hormones, and possibly dietary fiber.

Artherosclerosis—Prevention Begins at an Early Age

Most children found to have moderately elevated cholesterol levels have no evidence of a familial disorder or precipitating disease—diabetes, for example. Their elevated cholesterol levels are primarily related to an excessive intake of cholesterol or saturated fatty acids or both. The average cholesterol level in American children ranges anywhere from 50 to 100 mg/100 ml higher than levels in children from less developed countries who eat considerably less cholesterol containing foods and many fewer saturated fatty acids. Many people question the relationship of these higher cholesterol levels to the amount of milk consumed.

What are normal levels? The blood cholesterol level at birth is somewhere between 40 and 90 mg/100 ml with an average of about 60 to 70. It rises rather rapidly after birth into the 160 to 170 range by ages one to two years, and rises only slightly between ages two and twenty years, with average normal levels in American studies reported somewhere between 160 and 180. Many physicians feel that cholesterol levels should be kept in the range of 200 or lower; the previously accepted "normal" of 225 mg/100 ml is probably too high. It is interesting that when the sex glands are active, the level of cholesterol in women is lower than that in men. After the menopause, there is usually a sharp rise in the cholesterol level.

Although the type and amount of fat, as well as the cholesterol content of the diet, have usually been singled out as the culprits in high or elevated cholesterol levels, recent studies suggest that people with diets rich in fiber have lower cholesterol levels. In both animal and human studies, leguminous seeds, which are twice as rich as cereals in fiber content, appear to have a cholesterol-depressing effect. At any rate, vegetarians who have been studied show significantly lower cholesterol and triglyceride levels than those in the "control groups" consuming the usual American diet.

The exact mechanism by which atherosclerosis arises is not yet known, but it is clear that high blood cholesterol levels are associated with this disease process. There are, no doubt, many other contributing factors and, as you might expect when dealing with any subject where all the facts are not known, there are differences of opinion about all facets of the problem. For example, it is well known that egg yolks are high in cholesterol, but there is presently a great deal of controversy as to whether this cholesterol, when eaten, has a significant impact on blood cholesterol levels. The American Heart Association feels that caution is in order, however, and suggests that you not eat more than three egg yolks—the whites of eggs are not a problem—a week.

It is interesting that we never hear about the normal and necessary role cholesterol plays. One of its main functions is to facilitate the absorption of fatty acids, thus making them available as a source of energy. Cholesterol also gives rise to a substance from which vitamin D is formed by ultraviolet light when it penetrates the skin. The body makes enough cholesterol to supply these needs. Dietary cholesterol is not really required.

Triglyceride levels

Evidence is accumulating that raised blood triglycerides — the normal level is 50 to 150 mg/100 ml — place you at an increased risk of heart disese. So what are triglycerides?

Triglyceride is the form in which fats usually occur both in foodstuffs and in the fat deposits of animals. Eating a fatty meal will, therefore, raise your triglyceride level. Triglyceride levels can also be raised by eating carbohydrates. How?

Carbohydrates (that is, starches, cellulose, and sugar) when eaten, are ultimately converted into fat — triglycerides to be specific. Thus, after eating, the blood triglyceride level will increase. Not all carbohydrates raise triglyceride levels equally, however. Fructose, one of the components of ordinary table sugar, is more likely to raise triglyceride levels than others.

If you consistently eat a diet rich in carbohydrates, the blood triglyceride level will go up and will remain elevated — but usually for only a week or two. After that, the body appears to adapt to this type of diet and the triglyceride values start back down. The addition of polyunsaturated fats to the diet will also lower triglyceride levels.

It appears, therefore, that persistently high triglyceride levels are primarily the result of diets high in total calories and saturated fats and cholersterol. The large amount of sugar used by most Americans remains suspect since most diets that are high in saturated fats (as ours are) are also high in sugar intake, and we know that sugar raises triglyceride levels more readily than other carbohydrates. Obviously, the answers to this issue are only partially known.

Exercise

Regular physical exercise seems to protect against coronary heart disease, even in the presence of a diet that is typical of those found in populations where the incidence of atherosclerosis is high.

The typical diet leading to atherosclerosis is one high in saturated fats and cholesterol. Yet the Masai tribe in East Africa, who have extremely high intakes of saturated fats (their diet consists almost entirely of milk, meat, and blood from their cattle) have low blood cholesterol levels and rarely suffer from heart disease. This nomadic tribe is physically very active, however, walking great distances herding their cattle from place to place. Heredity may very well play an important part in this tribe's good health, but exercise is no doubt a very important factor as the following examples will show.

Other studies have shown that people in physically active jobs have less coronary heart disease, and that even when they do develop heart disease it

Artherosclerosis—Prevention Begins at an Early Age

is less severe and appears later in life than in people with physically inactive jobs. For example, London bus conductors, who have to scurry up and down the steps of their double-decker buses, have a lower incidence of heart disease than London bus drivers who remain seated. Likewise, letter carriers who must walk to deliver their letters have a lower incidence than telephone operators and post office clerks. Furthermore, when heart disease did strike the conductors and lettercarriers, it was less severe.

The American life-style has become more and more sedentary as prosperity and labor-saving devices have reduced the amount of manual labor required to earn a living and maintain a home. Along with these "advances" has come an increased incidence of heart disease. Other prosperous countries show the same pattern. The old adage, "with the good comes some bad," certainly applies here.

Overeating

Clearly, obesity not only aggravates cardiovascular diseases but also increases the likelihood of their development. Excessive weight overworks even a normal heart and circulatory system, let alone a damaged one. Add to this physical strain the excessive amounts of fat eaten and stored and the reduced exercise pattern of most obese people, and you have a blueprint for disaster.

For example, consider the mortality statistics. General mortality among obese men and women in the United States increases with each ten percent above ideal weight. Most of these deaths are a result of high blood pressure and coronary heart disease. Some day soon perhaps we will understand all the physiological and psychological factors involved in overeating and overweight.

Saturated fats

High intakes of saturated fats (discussed in detail in Chapter 2) are associated with elevated blood cholesterol and triglyceride levels and high death rates from coronary heart disease. A relatively high ratio of polyunsaturated fats to saturated fats often decreases these undesirable blood levels.

Most Americans obtain forty to forty-five percent of their daily calories from fats, with a large number of these calories coming from saturated fats. This intake is about ten percent too high, but of even more importance than the actual amount of fat eaten is the kind of fat eaten. The American Heart Association recommends that no more than ten percent of your daily fat allowance be from saturated fats.

Tension

It is difficult to say exactly what role the stress and strain of modern life plays in the development of atherosclerosis. There is no doubt, however, that once atherosclerosis is established, emotion can be the immediate cause of clinical symptoms.

One's blood cholesterol can even be noted to vacilate depending on emotional factors. For example, a person may have a high blood cholesterol level when under tension and, two weeks later, when on vacation and relaxed, have a normal blood level—even in the absence of any significant dietary change.

There is a behavior pattern described as Type A that is associated with increased risk of heart attacks. The Type A Personality is illustrated clearly by the *New Yorker* magazine cartoon that shows two middle-aged businessmen in shorts sitting on the porch of an expensive resort hotel. The one man says to the other, "If I were the type to relax, could I afford to be here?"

Smoking

Heart and vascular diseases, especially myocardial infarctions, occur much more frequently in heavy cigarette smokers than in those who do not smoke. In fact, cigarette smokers are from one and one-half to two and one-half times more likely to die from heart disease than nonsmokers. Heavy smokers have the highest death rate.

The "whys" of this relationship are not known: is it the vascular constriction action of nicotine, or is it that heavy smoking is typical of certain personality types and their reaction to stress is in question? We don't have the answers, but we do have the correlation!

The one main factor that influences whether or not a child starts smoking is the smoking behavior of those around him. The attitudes of parents are extremely important and are the major factors contributing to the life-style of an adolescent.

Hypertension

High blood pressure, which places increased demands on the coronary arteries, is thought to have several causes. A tendency toward high blood pressure is inheritable, with environmental factors probably playing an important role in the actual development of the problem. An excessive intake of salt is also felt to be a contributing factor. Some hypertensive patients are thin, but the incidence is much greater in persons who are obese. Also, recent research findings have shown that the presence or absence of certain mineral elements in the water may be an important factor. It has been observed that the incidence of atherosclerosis and coronary heart disease is lower in regions that have "hard" water. There are no explanations for many of these findings, but it is clear, nonetheless, that hypertension is associated with atherosclerosis.

What is your normal blood pressure? Blood pressure consists of two values: the systolic pressure—that occurring at the moment of the contraction of the left ventricle of the heart—and the diastolic pressure—that which exists as the ventricles fill with blood immediately before the next ventricular contraction occurs. The diastolic pressure is a more reliable guide to the presence or absence of hypertension than is the systolic pressure.

In healthy young adults, the systolic blood pressure is about 120 mm Hg and the diastolic pressure about 80 (usually spoken as "120 over 80" and written as "120/80"). There is usually a gradual rise in blood pressure as age advances and at 65 years the pressure is about 160/90.

Mild hypertension may be said to be present when the diastolic pressure is 90 to 105, moderate hypertension when the diastolic pressure is 105 to 120, and severe hypertension when the diastolic pressure exceeds 120.

Diabetes

Atherosclerosis occurs commonly and extensively in persons with diabetes. The impaired blood flow, thus, makes the person with diabetes more prone than others to gangrene of the toes and feet, to heart attacks, and to blindness. Strict control of the diabetic state offers the best chance of delaying the onset and progress of the vascular complications of diabetes. Diabetes is discussed in detail in a separate chapter.

In Summary

From various statistical data, we can draw a picture of the coronary-prone individual. He is a middle-aged male, is overweight, has a history of heart disease in his family, and has high blood pressure and elevated cholesterol and triglyceride levels. He smokes more than a pack of cigarettes a day, is hardworking but holds a stressful job requiring little physical exertion, and habitually eats food high in saturated fats and cholesterol.

Recommendations

Although heart transplantation or mechanical hearts may be possible in this day of scientific miracles, it is not possible to replace all the blood vessels that can get plugged up and lead to heart disease. Prevention is the answer. Practical preventive measures would include:
- Reduce saturated fat and cholesterol intake.
- Reduce calories for those who are overweight.
- Moderately increase intake of polyunsaturated fats.
- Maintain a good intake of protein, vitamins, and minerals.

TABLE 9
THE PRUDENT DIET
SUBSTITUTES FOR CHOLESTEROL-CONTAINING FOODS

Foods High in Cholesterol and/or Saturated Fats[1]	Recommended Substitutes[1]
Egg yolk	Egg white (no cholesterol or fat) Cholesterol-free egg substitute
Whole milk (6% SF by weight, 40% TC from SF, 30 mg cholesterol per 8 oz)	Skim milk (0.5% or less SF by weight, 7 mg cholesterol per 8 oz)
Cheeses (80% TC from fat, 60% TC from SF, 30 mg cholesterol per oz)	Whey cheeses, noncreamed cottage cheese
Butter (95% TC from fat, 60% TC from SF, 70 mg cholesterol per oz)	Soft corn oil or safflower oil margarines (no cholesterol, PF/SF ratio greater than 2)
Ice Cream (60% TC from fat, 30% TC from SF, 35 mg cholesterol per 1/2 cup)	Sherbets, nonsaturated fat ice milks
Fatty "marbled" red meats, hot dogs, hamburgers, luncheon meats, sausage, bacon (40-80% TC from fat, 20-50% TC from SF, 30-35 mg cholesterol per oz)	Limited amounts of lean red meats (30-40% TC from fat, 10-20% TC from SF, 30-35 mg cholesterol per oz)
Skin and internal organs, such as liver, kidney, brain (100-600 mg cholesterol per oz)	Fish and chicken (less SF and higher PF/SF ratio than lean red meat, 20 mg cholesterol per oz)
Shellfish (40-70 mg cholesterol per oz)	Textured vegetable protein products (no cholesterol low total fat content and high PF/SF ratio)

[1] The above values are approximates. Cholesterol is not found in vegetables, fruits, cereals or nuts. Some vegetable fats are naturally saturated (coconut, palm, cocoa); most vegetable fats are naturally polyunsaturated but all of them can be artifically saturated. Lean meats do not necessarily have less cholesterol but are lower in total fat and saturated fat content.

SF = saturated fat; PF = polyunsaturated fat; TC = total calories.

Source: Stare, Fredrick J., ed. *Atherosclerosis,* page 67. New York: MEDCOM, Inc., 1974.

- Place emphasis on more complex carbohydrates such as starches rather than sugars.
- Try to avoid undue emotional stress. Make time for leisure activities.
- Make exercise a part of your life-style.
- Eliminate, or at least reduce, cigarette smoking.
- Avoid excessive salt intakes.

Table 9 shows you ways to reduce the amount of saturated fats and cholesterol in your diet. Based on the evidence that we have thus far, these dietary changes should be instituted in childhood if we are to try and prevent the development of atherosclerosis. Once atherosclerosis is established, there is no evidence that it is reversible by dietary changes, but you can perhaps prevent its progression.

Federal regulations require labels to indicate nutritional composition if the foods are enriched or fortified or if a nutritional claim is made for the food. Other foods are not required to be so labeled. Many companies have started voluntarily including this type of information on their products' labels. This trend indicates a definite concern for the health of the American people and should be commended and further encouraged, although an educational program will probably be necessary for this information to be understood and useful to consumers. Unfortunately, cholesterol is not one of the items usually listed, nor does the label tell you how much of the product's fat content is in the form of saturated fatty acids.

Diabetes

What Is Diabetes?

Diabetes is a disease that results in the body being unable to use food properly. Most authorities agree that the tendency to develop diabetes is inherited although, in the majority of cases, diabetes doesn't "start" until middle-age. The way in which diabetes is transmitted is still uncertain, as there are no specific genetic "markers."

There are other factors that also play a role in the likelihood of developing diabetes: pregnancy, infections, physical injury, or severe emotional stress. The association between obesity and diabetes has also long been recognized, but it is not clear whether obesity is the result or the cause of diabetes. However, it is becoming increasingly more apparent that the diabetes associated with obesity can be controlled by weight loss. This appears to be true even for those persons falling in the upper ranges of the so-called desirable weight. Diabetes is also occasionally seen as a result of other diseases and/or treatments.

Diabetes can start at any age although, as mentioned above, it is primarily a disease of middle age—often referred to as *maturity-onset diabetes*. In fact, four out of five persons with diabetes are forty-five years old or over. *Early-onset* or *juvenile* diabetes usually begins before the age of 15 years. Both the symptoms and the treatment vary with the age of onset. This will be discussed later in the chapter; first, let's take a look at what happens normally when we eat. During digestion, much of the food is changed into a form of sugar called *glucose*. This glucose is then carried to the various parts of the body by the bloodstream for use as energy and for body maintenance. If not all of the glucose is needed immediately, it is changed into still another form of sugar called *glycogen*. This glycogen is stored in the liver and muscles to be used whenever there is a demand for energy. When the body needs it, the glycogen is changed back into glucose and released into the bloodstream for use.

The body cannot use the glucose or store it (in the form of glycogen) without the aid of a hormone produced by the pancreas called *insulin*. When the pancreas fails to produce an adequate supply of insulin, or when the insulin cannot be used properly, glucose cannot be used or stored in the body and, thus, the glucose accumulates in the bloodstream, causing blood sugar levels to rise above normal; this state is called *hyperglycemia*. When the amount of sugar in the blood reaches a certain level, the glucose passes through the kidneys and "spills" into the urine. And this is extactly the problem that diabetics have: not enough or a poor use of insulin and, therefore, glucose in the urine and abnormally large amounts of glucose in the blood. So, what happens with all this excess glucose? A number of things; let's take them one by one.

1. When there is a large amount of glucose in the blood, water is pulled out of the body's tissues and, consequently, the person has to urinate more often than usual. The body then demands that these fluids be replaced, resulting in excessive thirst.

2. Since much of the food that is eaten cannot be used or stored for energy — because there isn't enough insulin available — the diabetic often becomes weak and tired. And even though there is an increase in appetite and in the amount of food eaten, there is frequently a loss of body weight.

3. In an attempt to supply energy — because of the problem mentioned above — the body breaks down available fat and protein. In the process, ketone bodies (beta-hydroxybutyrate, acetoacetate, and acetone) are formed. When these substances (which can be used as an alternate energy source) are produced faster than the body can eliminate them, they accumulate and act as poisons in the body. This accumulation is called *acidosis* or *ketosis*.

When acidosis or ketosis occurs, the body goes all out to try and neutralize the acid bodies by combining them with the alkaline reserves normally present in the blood. Even more fluids are needed to wash out the acids. This causes increased thirst and an increase in the production of urine. Eventually, the tissue fluids are exhausted, and the body become dehydrated. If this continues, the diabetic becomes unconscious and goes into coma. Untreated coma can lead to death.

4. Muscular activity burns up glucose and can, therefore, help the diabetic get rid of the excessive amounts of glucose in the blood. However, too much exercise can use up large amounts of glucose and cause a sharp drop in the blood sugar level, producing a state called *hypoglycemia*. When the blood sugar level falls too low, the brain cannot operate at full efficiency, and fatigue, headache, drowsiness, nervousness, and many other serious symptoms may appear. The blood sugar level must be restored to normal so that the brain can function normally.

How do children with diabetes differ from adults with diabetes? Whereas the adult usually has a gradual onset of the disease, the onset of symptoms in children is often quite sudden and usually represents a more severe type of diabetes. They are thirsty, drink large quantities of fluid, and void larger amounts of urine frequently. The child may rapidly lose weight and become weak. They are often undernourished by the time the condition is diagnosed. Additionally, children's blood sugar levels change more easily than adults' and, thus, both hyperglycemia (too much glucose) and hypoglycemia (too little glucose) occur more readily. Also, patterns of physical activity are less consistent in children; emotional factors, particularly during adolescence, are likely to influence the course of the disease, and the child is more likely to suffer from various infections which can easily throw him or her into acidosis with very little warning.

How Is it Treated?

The treatment for diabetes is a very individualized thing, and depends not only on the extent of the person's insulin deficiency but also on his or her general physical condition and life-style. In general, however, the underlying principle of dietary therapy of the adult-onset patient with diabetes is the correction of the body weight; the person needs to restrict his or her caloric intake. On the other hand, the underlying dietary therapy of the juvenile-onset patient with diabetes is constancy of food content on a day-to-day basis, coupled with relatively frequent intervals of feeding. Let's look at each of the components of therapy.

Diet

Dietary requirements differ with the individual, the severity of the disease, the type and amount of insulin received, and the amount of exercise. To understand the reasoning behind the dietary measures prescribed by the physician, we need to look again briefly at the basic problem in diabetics: the inability to use foods properly. Let's look first at the kinds of food we eat.

As you will recall, foods are a combination of proteins, fats, and carbohyrdates. The typical diet contains about 12 percent protein, 38 percent fat, and 50 percent carbohydrates. Carbohydrates (sugar, starches, fiber) are readily converted to glucose for use as energy. Proteins also provide a supply of potential glucose, but their conversion to glucose is a very gradual affair and actually occurs to a much lesser extent than with carbohydrates — except when the supply of carbohydrates is greatly reduced. Fats may serve as an alternate energy source after further metabolism. Thus, proteins and fats are not as likely to cause a sudden increase in the blood sugar level as are the

The Commonsense Guide to Good Eating

carbohydrates. To a large degree, therefore, dietary control revolves around regulation of the amount of carbohydrates eaten.

As you might expect, not only must the type of food eaten be regulated but so must the time at which it is eaten. A meal skipped or delayed too long can upset the diabetic's delicate body chemistry. Likewise, if the intake of food varies from day to day it is impossible to work out a steady insulin or other drug therapy to cover it.

To simplify food identification (that is, knowing whether the food is mainly made up of carbohydrates, proteins, or fats) while providing the diabetic maximum flexibility in choosing what to eat, a system of food exchanges or substitutions is used. This is a system wherein foods are grouped according to their food value. Each food in any one list contains approximately the same number of calories and the same amount of protein, fat, and carbohydrates as any other food on that same list. Thus, one of these foods can be exchanged or substituted for another on the same list—hence, the name Exchange or Substitution Lists. Dietary prescriptions are usually given in terms of how many exchanges or substitutions are allowed each day from each list. This method of dietary control has also proven to be very effective in weight regulation, a concern of our population in general and diabetics in particular. The exchange lists are given in Chapter 9, Diet Plans.

Maintaining body weight at or slightly below the statistical desirable weight is of critical importance to the person with diabetes. Weight greatly influences the amount of drugs necessary to control the diabetic's clinical condition. As a matter of fact, it is often a weight gain that triggers the development of symptoms in maturity-onset diabetes.

Insulin therapy

There are many types of insulin available. They differ primarily in how fast they work and how long the effects last. Insulin cannot be taken by mouth because it is destroyed by the digestive juices. Juvenile diabetics almost always require insulin injections, while the adult can be treated by diet alone or by a combination of diet and oral medications.

Despite some earlier suggestions in the literature, oral hypoglycemics should not be used in juvenile-onset diabetes because these patients lack insulin production and require insulin administration. There is presently a great deal of controversy about the entire subject of oral agents.

Periods of stress such as illness, injury, or pregnancy may alter the individual's need for insulin. Insulin helps the body use its store of glucose more effectively, thus preventing a buildup of the glucose in the blood.

Exercise

Regular exercise plays an important role in the management of diabetes.

Diabetes

Besides helping to burn up glucose, exercise apparently causes an increased sensitivity to insulin action and, thus, may actually decrease the amount of insulin or other antidiabetic medication needed. Wide variations in exercise patterns from day to day or weekday to weekend should be avoided or, if not avoided, clearly planned for. With strenuous exercise one day and little or no exercise the next, the diabetic's blood sugar level is apt to be too low the first day and too high the following day. Such fluctuations require an adjustment in the amount of food eaten.

When strenuous exercise is called for, such as in many sports, 10 gram carbohydrate snacks may be required every thirty to forty-five minutes during the period of intense exercise. This will usually prevent hypoglycemia. There is no need for the person with diabetes to avoid active sports. Proper diet and medication adjustments usually allow the diabetic to participate comfortably. There are a number of professional athletes who have diabetes.

Urine testing

The measurement of glucose (sugar) in the urine is one way to monitor how well the diet, insulin, and exercise are balanced. If there is a marked change in the glucose, some adjustment may be necessary. Another reason for urine testing is to see if there is acetone (ketone bodies) in the urine. The presence of acetone may warn of impending acidosis which could lead to diabetic coma if untreated.

Testing the urine for either glucose or acetone is a very easy procedure. Specially treated strips are dipped into the urine. The color that the strip turns is an indication of how much glucose or acetone is present. There are also special tablets which are used for this purpose.

Complications

The two most common short-term complications of diabetes are hypoglycemia (low blood sugar) and acidosis. Hypoglycemic reactions have a rapid onset, usually within minutes or a few hours. Acidosis, leading to diabetic coma, develops gradually over a few hours or days. It is very important to distinguish between the two conditions because the treatment for one is entirely different from the treatment for the other. Hypoglycemia is easily corrected if treated immediately. Acidosis is more difficult to control. Long-term complications include blood vessel disease, especially of the eyes and kidneys, and diseases of the central nervous system.

Special Dietary Problems

Food Allergies

Approximately one in every ten persons suffers from some sort of allergy. Food allergies account for only a small portion of this number, but for those so afflicted it is a serious problem.

Allergies can be described as abnormal reactions by an individual to the food he or she eats, the air he or she breathes, or to the substances he or she touches. A predisposition to allergy can definitely be inherited, although not all potentially allergic individuals develop clear allergies.

Allergic patterns vary from person to person, and even change with age. Some individuals become sensitive to certain foods at an early age, some not until later in life. Some food allergies are accompanied by inhalant allergies such as to dust, pollen, animal hair and dander, while some food allergies disappear about the time inhalant allergies appear. It's a complicated picture and problem, as you can see.

An allergic reaction may occur almost immediately after eating the offending food or it may be delayed hours or even days. The reaction can take many forms—runny nose and red eyes, headache, skin rash, bad breath, stomach pain and diarrhea, wheezing, etc.—although for any one individual the reaction is usually the same each time the food is encountered.

Some individuals are only mildly sensitive and can eat a particular food for several days without trouble, whereas others have violent reactions within minutes after eating even minute amounts of the offending food.

Many food allergies go unrecognized unless a detailed food diary is kept over a period of several weeks. This record of food intake an unpleasant symptoms gives you a better chance to correlate the two, especially when the reaction is a delayed one. Keep in mind, however, that foods that offend in their raw state may not offend when cooked. Thus, many people allergic to raw or pasturized milk can easily tolerate milk when it is boiled as in sauces, cakes, etc.

If you have a definite food allergy, it is important for you and your doctor to know about it. Many therapeutic or immunizing solutions for injections are prepared using a food base and could, thus, result in a severe or even fatal reaction if given to a person highly sensitive to that particular food.

The most common food offenders are: wheat, milk, eggs (particularly egg yolks), seafood (especially shellfish), chocolate, corn, nuts, tomatoes, oranges, chicken, pork, and some spices. Chemical irritation of the skin when eating oranges should not be confused with allergy. Foods rarely causing problems are rice, lamb, gelatin, peaches, pears, carrots, lettuce, artichokes, sesame oil, and apples.

Lactose Intolerance

Medical literature in the last few years has revealed an almost international prevalence of the human being's limited ability to digest a large amount of lactose ("lactose intolerance"), the main carbohydrate in milk ("milk sugar") which enhances mineral and protein utilization. Symptoms usually occur thirty to ninety minutes after ingestion, and range from abdominal distention and mild discomfort to cramps and diarrhea. Black persons and Orientals are particularly susceptible.

Nutrient utilization in lactose intolerant subjects has not differed significantly from that in normal subjects, however. Recent studies have revealed that lactose intolerance does not denote milk intolerance. It has been demonstrated that individuals with a limited ability to digest lactose can consume nutritionally useful quantities of milk. Also, milk products such as yogurt and cheese, in which some of the lactose has been broken down by bacterial fermentation, can often be consumed without discomfort.

Lactose intolerance is not an allergy but rather a result of an enzyme deficiency.

Acne

Exactly what causes acne is not clearly understood. Many dermatologists feel that acne is associated with increases in certain hormones—which are secreted in increasing amounts during adolescence—that effect the sebaceous glands. These glands produce an oily substance called sebum which helps prevent skin dryness. Problems arise when something—such as blackheads—blocks the gland opening, thereby interfering with normal flow of sebum. Bacteria then invade the area, and the area may become inflamed and infected.

Acne is not caused by sexual activity—either too much or too little! Nor

Special Dietary Problems

is there any proven association of this disorder with nutritional deficiency or as a reaction to specific foods, though at one time or another almost every food imaginable has been accused of causing or aggravating acne. If you feel that certain foods aggravate your problems, by all means try eliminating them from your diet for a few weeks and see if your skin condition improves. More than likely, however, you'll find that keeping your skin and hair clean (although acne is not caused by dirty skin), avoiding greasy skin preparations, not "picking," and using a clean pillowcase each night will be more effective than dietary intervention. Over-the-counter preparations containing sulfur, benzoyl peroxide, resorcinol, or salicylic acid may also prove helpful.

Who will get acne? Almost everyone will have acne before reaching adulthood, but only a small percentage of those affected will have severe problems. For those unfortunate few, however, medical attention is clearly called for to help prevent pitting and scarring. This is not a time for do-it-yourself remedies or waiting for it "to go away" with age.

Dental Health

"The teeth are a living memorial to the defects of the previous diet. Too often by middle age a few crumbling and unstable tombstones are all that remain to commemorate past errors."[1]

The life of a tooth begins long before birth, while the baby is still being formed. Successful tooth development is, therefore initially dependent on the adequacy of the mother's nutrition. For the continuation of tooth formation after birth, the baby must still rely on the mother to provide the proper nutrients, either from her own body stores by way of breast feeding or by "formula" supplementation. Critical to the development of healthy teeth resistant to decay are: calcium, phosphorus, fluorine, and vitamins A, C, and D.

A calcium-phosphorus balance is required to form the hard structure of the teeth. Vitamin D is essential as it aids in the absorption and utilization of calcium and phosphorus. Vitamin A is necessary to the normal development of epithelial cells, the cells from which tooth enamel has its origin. Vitamin C is required for the formation of the connective tissue which holds the cells together. Deposits of fluorine in the teeth protect them against decay.

Healthy gums, firmly attached to the teeth, are essential for good oral health and comfort. Periodontal disease, wherein the gum falls away from the teeth and infection sets in, is quite painful. There is a correlation between accumulations of tartar at the base of the teeth and periodontal disease.

In this country, dental ill health is probably related more to faulty eating habits and inadequate oral hygiene than to poor nutrition. Sticky carbohydrates such as white bread and candy, when not removed promptly from the teeth, provide an excellent breeding ground for the bacteria to start the work that leads to cavities. Diets consisting largely of soft foods, combined with inadequate brushing and flossing of the teeth, allow tartar to accumulate at a surprising rate.

Considerable clinical and experimental evidence indicates that erosion, etching, or decalcification of calcified tooth structure may be produced not only by injudicious consumption of lemon juice but by other highly acidic carbonated beverages, liquids, or medicines if the acids, organic or inorganic, are of low enough pH.

Fluorine plays an important role in preventing tooth decay and, hence, in most parts of this country this element is added to our public water supply. Some localities have no need of fluorine addition since their water already contains adequate amounts of this mineral. Yet other areas have the problem of an excess of fluorine occuring naturally in their water supply. If the drinking water contains more than two parts fluorine per million parts water, white flecks may appear in the tooth enamel, whereas concentrations of five parts fluorine per million parts water may result in an uneven and brown-stained enamel surface. Though these teeth are still resistant to dental decay, they are not attractive and an alternative drinking source such as bottled water may be desired. Your dentist or local city or county health department can advise you about the fluorine content of your particular water supply.

There is still much confusion about the various factors involved in tooth decay and its prevention. Many fears about fluoridation are based on scanty and incorrect knowledge. There is still much need for public education. Fluorine is further discussed in The Whys and Wherefores of Vitamins and Minerals in the Appendix.

Our nation's dental bill is staggering — over four billion dollars a year — yet it is estimated that one out of every five Americans will need dentures by the age of forty-five. Early attention to preventive measures are necessary if we are to reverse this most unpleasant trend.

Companies and agencies providing pre-paid medical insurance plans should be urged to extend their coverage to include routine dental examinations and treatment. And it is imperative that we do something about providing free dental care for families with reduced incomes. It makes no sense to provide free breakfasts and lunches if the children aren't going to have any teeth with which to eat them!

Pregnancy

Pregnancy is the leading reason why teenage girls leave school before graduation. Two percent of all teenage births are to mothers under fifteen years

Special Dietary Problems

of age; this means almost 10,000 babies born to girls not yet grown themselves. Births to teenage mothers account for 17 percent of all births in the United States. The birth represents a first child for 77 percent of the teenagers, a second child for 18 percent, and a third or more child for 4 percent.

Late and irregular prenatal care is, unfortunately, characteristic of pregnant adolescents. Add to this lack of nutritional or any other guidance the emotional stress many of these youngsters face, and a sizable problem surfaces. Not only does the very young teenage mother run increased risks of complications of pregnancy, the baby does not fare so well either. Premature delivery is not uncommon, and these babies face a greater chance of death or deformity than infants born to women at older ages.

Older teenage mothers do not seem to suffer unduly from pregnancy complications, but their babies still show lower birth weights and increased risk of death or abnormalities. Whether or not the lower birth weights of children born to teenage mothers are attributable to the double nutritional stress of the mother's own adolescent growth plus that of her baby, is not known. It has been claimed, however, that adolescent girls in the United States usually have poorer diets than the rest of the members of a family. This is thought to be true for all socio-economic groups, though it appears to be worse in the lower socio-economic families.

As you might expect, obese women have more problems during pregnancy than those of normal weight. Interestingly enough, however, markedly underweight mothers also have a higher incidence of preeclampsia (severe high blood pressure, sometimes accompanied by convulsions) than normal weight mothers.

Regular prenatal care is necessary, regardless of the pregnant woman's age, to insure the mother and baby the safest pregnancy and delivery possible. Most areas have clinics with a sliding professional fee scale, so that the cost is adjusted depending on the recipient's ability to pay. There is no excuse for not getting prenatal care under any circumstances, for there are many community and state agencies available to advise and help those in need.

Eating for two? There are special nutritional requirements during pregnancy, but if you unduly increase your caloric intake in the mistaken notion that you must eat enough for two, chances are you will still look like two long after you are just one!

Caloric requirements during pregnancy are best evaluated by your physician depending on your pre-pregnancy weight, general health, and activity level. Physicians no longer seem to be quite as strict about weight gained during pregnancy as they were even just a few years ago, but there are so many variables that could critically influence the amount of weight *you* should gain that you should really seek and adhere to your doctor's advice.

The Commonsense Guide to Good Eating

Anemia due to iron deficiency is common during and after pregnancy because of the large amount of iron given over to the fetus and enveloping placenta and because of the extra needs to increase red blood cell volume. A diet rich in iron is necessary to protect the mother; it is also required so that the baby will be born with a liver well stored with iron to see him or her over the early months after birth when his or her diet will consist mainly of milk, a food low in iron content.

Even for a healthy woman with a good diet, the provision of enough milk to meet the needs of a vigorous infant is a physiological strain. When the mother's diet is inadequate, she will probably continue to supply milk, but her own stores of nutrients will be drawn upon and evidence of maternal malnutrition may well appear. This physiological stress is often made even worse by the physical and emotional requirements of tending for a new baby. The pale, chronically fatigued new mother is an altogether too common sight. Continued concern for the mother's health is called for, in addition to post-natal guidance in the care of her infant.

Formation of the baby's teeth begins in the last half of pregnancy and continues after birth. Extra calcium for the mother during pregnancy and when breast feeding will give the baby his or her best chance for healthy teeth and bones. There is no proof that significant decalcification of the mother's teeth occurs during pregnancy. Dental decay is not more frequent than normal, despite the old saying of "a tooth for each baby."

Doctors often prescribe vitamin and mineral supplements to be taken during pregnancy and breast feeding to ensure the mother's and baby's nutritional well-being. Self-determination of nutrient requirements is not a wise idea at this critical period in your life and in the life of your baby. Also, remember when taking these supplements that just because a little may be good, a lot is not necessarily better; the doctor's instructions should always be followed closely.

Don't delude yourself into thinking that you can neglect your nutritional well-being until the time of pregnancy. Studies show that the health and birth weight of the infant is more related to the mother's long-term diet habits than to her diet while pregnant. A long history of adequate nutrition better prepares the mother and the baby for pregnancy than does a poor nutritional history followed by an attempt to correct the mother's diet while pregnant.

Many pregnant women find that a number of small meals rather than three large ones helps prevent indigestion and heartburn, especially in the later months of pregnancy when the uterus is substantially enlarged. Smaller meals are usually also better tolerated if the mother is suffering from nausea "Morning sickness," often seen in early pregnancy, can sometimes be avoided if the mother will slowly eat a snack of dry toast and crackers while still in bed, ten to fifteen minutes before arising.

Constipation is not uncommon during pregnancy. If this is a problem, small amounts of figs, prune juice, or stewed prunes will probably help. Laxatives should not be taken during pregnancy unless so advised by your physician.

Diet and Physical Training Programs

Before undertaking a strenuous training program of any kind, it is important to assess your present physical condition. It is folly to rush from extreme inactivity to extreme activity whether it be tennis, football, or cycling. Some limbering up and muscle toning exercises would be a wise first step, especially as one advances in age. A talk with your physician and a "stress" electrocardiogram (EKG) should be considered for anyone with a personal or close-family history of heart disease.

If you are just embarking on a training program, you may find that even though you increase your caloric intake to meet your higher energy needs, you may lose weight. Interestingly enough, however, underweight people usually gain weight when training begins. Our bodies seem to strive toward a lean firm appearance, and exercise coupled with adequate nutrition is clearly the key.

During strenuous training there is an increased need to assure adequate protein and iron intake to build muscles and prevent anemia. Thiamin (vitamin B_1) also becomes more important because increasing exercise causes faster utilization of this vitamin. Athletes with a thiamin deficiency usually perform less well than those with an adequate supply; excessive intakes are definitely not called for, however, nor will they be of additional value. Vitamin and mineral supplements can be used if your supply from foods is inadequate, but these supplements will not provide your protein requirements.

Whether to eat or not before an athletic event has been asked repeatedly over the years, and tests have been conducted to measure the effect of various diets on performance. The answer depends on a number of considerations: whether the athletic event is of long or short duration, how strenuous the activity is, and how the individual responds to the tension and physical stress of competition.

In events lasting no more than one hour, a regular meal two or three hours before should adequately provide the necessary energy and cause no problems. However, although protein is needed to build muscles and repair cells, many seasoned coaches and athletes feel that protein is not the food of choice prior to competition. What is needed at this point is food that can be quickly converted into energy, and carbohydrates do this well.

In events lasting several hours, a great number of calories of energy may be expended; for example, a racing bicyclist many use up 600 calories an hour. The body's store of carbohydrates and fats can cope with only part of this excessive energy expenditure; some other easily assimilated food — sugar — should be taken during the event. This extra energy intake is best taken in small amounts at frequent intervals since large quantities, though rapidly absorbed, may not be immediately available to the muscles.

Even a minor degree of dehydration impairs muscle efficiency. Fluid and salt losses through sweating are a problem when there is continued high energy output. In short-term sports, salt loss is not usually a problem (unless it is very hot) and the fluid can be replaced by water or a sweetened drink. When salt needs to be replaced as well as water, some form of carbohydrate should be taken at the same time since carbohydrates improve salt absorption. Sweetened beverages, hard candy, dried fruits, or jelly can be combined with 0.2 percent salt solution or salted crackers or chips to accomplish this purpose.

Coffee and tea prior to competitive events are best avoided unless you are thoroughly used to drinking these mild stimulants. Alcohol, though not harmful during training when taken in small amounts and by people accustomed to its use, greatly impairs judgment and coordination — even taken in small quantities — and so should be avoided before athletic events.

Most school and community physical education programs concentrate on the individual who is already in pretty good physical condition. There needs to be a stepped-up effort to provide greater and more routine opportunities for obese or otherwise handicapped people also to improve their physical activity pattern. Programs should not be so oriented toward team participation; if people are to continue to exercise in later years, skills and interest must be developed in activities that can be persued on a more individual basis — such as golfing, tennis, swimming, cycling.

Achievement for the Poor

The most basic human need relates to hunger and thirst. Assuring that every child has enough to eat has to precede any expectation for learning. Too often, however, school feeding is viewed as extraneous to education and is among the earlier programs to be considered for cut-back when funds are short.

When extreme hunger is the normal condition, one cannot expect a positive approach to other aspects of living. Just as a hungry child cannot concentrate in school, the hungry adult cannot be a productive worker. If the cycle is not broken, the gap between the "haves" and the "have nots" in a society will widen.

When looking at the dollars available to the poor, it is well to remember that a large percentage of the amount must go for food—especially at today's prices. Yet, ill-equipped kitchens, fatigue, and frequent ill health all combine to make the more expensive convenience foods even more important to the poor than to the prosperous.

One must also remember that the poor are exposed to the same inducements to buy as are all Americans, so that priorities are sometimes hard to set. The problems of the poor are complex and they are not the same for all individuals. The poor are not a homogeneous group. They differ from each other psychologically, culturally, and ethnically, as well as in the degree of their poverty, the reasons for it, and the length of time they have been poor.

The poor deserve respect for the many solutions to their own problems that they have resolved for themselves. Building on current practices is a more effective way to induce change than is criticism which is bound to arouse resentment.

Increasing the Quality of Life for the Elderly and the Chronically Ill

Individuals over sixty-five years of age represent almost ten percent of the population of the United States—approximately twenty million people. This age group is increasing in numbers more rapidly than is the population at large. Census experts predict that by the year 2000, at least thirty million people in the United States will be sixty-five or older—and this is assuming that significant breakthroughs in the treatment and prevention of cancer and cardiovascular-renal diseases do not occur!

One of the major problems of the elderly with regard to obtaining an adequate diet is low income. The poor and the elderly represent widely overlapping groups in our population. Another problem relates to chronic illness. It is estimated that three-fourths of the noninstitutional population over sixty-five have one or more chronic conditions, and that almost two out of five have a chronic condition that limits their activity.

Caloric needs decrease with age owing to reduced basal metabolic rate and reduced physical activity, without an appreciable decrease in the need for protein, vitamins, and minerals. This may make the elderly person vulnerable to nutrient deficiency. Additionally, as people grow older they may lose the motivation to apply the knowledge that they already have. Thus, attempts to improve nutrition must include efforts to improve the individual's desire to help himself or herself as well as to provide accurate nutrition information.

The Commonsense Guide to Good Eating

There are increasing efforts to improve the quality of the older person's life rather than just aiming for longevity. Early preventive nutritional practices may help ward off some of the problems of illness associated with heart and other diseases, but continuing good nutrition should also be a part of the campaign.

Food Poisoning

Words of Warning

Food poisoning may result from bacteria or their products, parasite infestation, chemical contamination, or naturally occurring toxins. Food allergies are not usually included under the category food poisoning because the food ingested is wholesome—it is the indivdual's reaction to the food that is abnormal.

Though food poisoning may result from a variety of causes, there is a tendency for people to use the blanket term *ptomaine poisoning. Ptomaine* comes from the word *ptoma,* meaning "corpse." In other words, there is a tendency to associate food poisoning with food that is rotten. However, rotting food does not necessarily give rise to toxic substances involved in food poisoning. Limburger cheese contains decomposing organic matter, yet it is a perfectly safe food. Many peoples of the world actually consider certain rotten foods a delicacy. Eskimos in Greenland eat rotten seal meat and fish, the Samoyedes use rotten fish, and the Chinese serve rotten eggs.

All of this is not to say that all rotten foods are safe, but rather to point out that the common assumption that a food must be rotten to be poisonous is not true. On the contrary, most cases of food poisoning result from bacterial contamination of food that often changes neither the looks, smell, nor taste of the infected food.

Let's look more closely at each of the different causes of food poisoning.

Bacteria or Their Products

Bacteria or their products are responsible for the majority of food poisoning incidents. Certain of these microorganisms are so common that the chances for food contamination are very high. For example, it has been estimated that about one-half the population carries staphylococci organisms in the throat or on the skin. Strict sanitary precautions are required to keep such bacteria under control. The foods involved in bacterial food poisoning are usually those that provide a good breeding ground for the specific organism, as you will see in the following descriptions of causative agents.

Botulism

Botulism, the most deadly of the foodborne poisonings, is due to toxins formed by the growth of botulinum microorganisms which are commonly found in the soil. The term *botulism* is derived from a word meaning "sausage" and was coined by German physicians at the beginning of the nineteenth century, probably because the poisoning was sometimes seen in persons who had eaten contaminated sausage.

Botulinum bacteria grow only in the absence of air, thus making canned food from which air is excluded ideal for the growth of these dangerous organisms. The botulism bacteria will not grow in an acid medium, therefore, the majority of cases of botulism come from eating non-acid foods such as beets, corn, and string beans.

In the canning process, boiling alone is not enough to assure complete sterilization of low-acid foods. Temperatures of 249°F or more for ten to fifteen minutes are required to destroy the botulinum spore. Though there have been deaths from contaminated commercially processed foods, this is relatively uncommon as they are usually cooked at high temperatures. Most instances of botulinus poisoning are caused by the ingestion of improperly prepared home-preserved non-acid foods.

Symptoms of botulism usually appear with 12 to 36 hours. The earliest symptom is usually fatigue, sometimes associated with dizziness or headache. Double-vision is an early occurrence. The tongue is usually coated and swollen, and there is difficulty in swallowing and speaking. Medical care is urgently required for the early administration of the specific antitoxin to prevent a serious illness and/or death.

Prevention of botulism depends on careful examination of food, watching for abnormal taste, odor, gas (don't buy any canned food with a swollen puffy top — this could signal the presence of gas inside the can), sediment, or softening. It should be kept in mind, however, that there may be no observable alteration in the food. Foods contaminated with the botulinum toxin frequently have a rancid or bad odor or taste, but this is sometimes difficult to detect. So when in doubt throw the food away. Don't taste it "to be sure" — you may not live to tell your tale. When possible, home-canned products should be cooked for fifteen minutes before using.

Clostridium perfringens

Clostridium perfringens is present in soil, water, milk, dust, sewage, and the intestinal canal of man and animals and is rapidly supplanting toxin-producing staphylococci as the most common cause of food poisoning in this country. These organisms are more heat resistant than staphylococci and are, therefore, more difficult to control.

Clostridium perfringens grow best from 85 to 115°F and thus, the typical picture is one of diarrhea with abdominal pain developing eight to 24 hours after the ingestion of food stored at a warm temperature for several hours after cooking. Meat and meat products such as gravy, creamed chicken, stew, or soup are the usual offenders. Recovery is usually uneventful in 12 to 24 hours.

Salmonella

Salmonella strains, long associated with food poisoning, gain entrance to the human body in food that becomes infected. Sources of the poisoning include meat from sick animals, raw or improperly pasteurized milk, infected frozen eggs or egg powder products, foods contaminated by flies or sick rats, and last but not least human carriers. By-products of the meat packing industry—bone meal, fertilizer, and pet foods—may constitute an important means by which salmonellosis is spread.

Salmonella are widespread in nature, and readily increase in number under favorable conditions of time and temperature. Since the size of the infecting dose of bacteria bears a close relationship to the speed of onset of symptoms and to the severity of the illness, danger arises from bacterial multiplication. Outbreaks of salmonella poisoning are especially likely to occur whenever large amounts of food are prepared and when the remaining food not consumed is kept for future meals. The danger of infection is greatly increased if such food is kept at a warm temperature instead of being stored in a refrigerator.

The types of food that are particularly likely to be infected are twice-cooked meat dishes, stews, gravies, soups, custards, milk and synthetic cream; also canned foods which, although usually initially sterile, may become infected if not consumed immediately after the can has been opened. Chicken and turkey dressing provide an *excellent* breeding ground because the poultry cavity may be a good insulator. Unless sufficient time and temperature in cooking are allowed, salmonella in the center of the stuffing may not be destroyed and may, in fact multiply. By the same token, poultry should not be refrigerated with the stuffing left inside because the cold may not adequately penetrate the stuffing.

The onset of symptoms varies from 72 hours after the contaminated food has been eaten. Headache and chills may be the initial symptoms. These are usually followed by abdominal cramps and persistent, foul-smelling diarrhea which may become very watery and green. Nausea, vomiting, fever, prostration, muscle weakness, faintness, and thirst are usually present. Also noted are restlessness, muscle twitching, drowsiness, and "fever blisters." Symptomatic treatment should include restriction of food intake to liquids and bland, soft solids. Antibiotic therapy is called for only when the infection is severe and correctly diagnosed by stool cultures.

Sanitation is the key to control of this infection. Meat and eggs should be adequately cooked; water and milk supplies controlled; fresh foods properly handled; and carriers treated and eliminated as food handlers.

Staphylococcus

Staphylococcus food poisoning is produced by a toxin (a poisonous substance) formed in the food before ingestion. It is the most common type of all food poisonings in the United States, involving almost everyone at one time or another. The conditions necessary for an outbreak of staphylococcus food poisoning are contamination of a food with toxin-producing staphylococci; a suitable food in which the organism can grow; and keeping the food for a sufficient time at a temperature compatible with growth (at or above room temperature for several hours).

A wide variety of foods have been implicated in this type of poisoning including milk, cheese, ice cream, cream-filled bakery goods, tongue, rapid-cured hams, chicken or potato salad, dried beef, sausage, and chicken gravy. Usually there is a history of the food having been kept warm for several hours before being served. Foods may also be contaminated from infected food handlers since staphylococci are common organisms found in the throats of individuals, on their skin, and in great abundance in the postnasal drip of persons recovering from colds.

Symptoms usually appear within three hours after eating. The incubation period is influenced both by the amount of toxin consumed and the susceptibility of the individual. The first symptom observed is usually salivation, followed by nausea, vomiting, retching, abdominal cramps, prostration, and diarrhea. Symptoms of shock have also been observed. As a rule, acute symptoms are of short duration and generally subside after five to six hours. A few fatal cases have occurred, usually in the very young, the aged, or the debilitated.

In staphylococcus food poisoning, vomiting and diarrhea are generally severe enough to free the gastrointestinal tract of the toxin without the use of a stomach pump. The individual will need to be given fluids to replace those lost, but no specific drug or serum therapy is of value.

The best control of staphylococcal food poisoning consists of adequate refrigeration of perishable foods, thereby making conditions unfavorable for the production of the toxin. It should be kept in mind that heat will kill the staphylococci but usually does not destroy the toxin the staphylococci have produced.

Food Poisoning

Streptococcus

Streptococcus faecalis is a natural inhabitant of the intestinal tract of man and animals and, as a consequence, is in man's food and drink. However, unusually large numbers of this bacteria may lead to an outbreak of streptococcus food poisoning, with the number of bacteria ingested playing a role both in speed of onset and severity of symptoms.

Streptococcus faecalis is characterized by its ability to grow fairly rapidly over a wide temperature range. Consequently it lurks in a variety of foods, especially cream-filled pastries, dressings in meat and fowl, and canned foods or leftovers that have not been recooked.

The incubation period from the time of eating the contaminated food to the onset of illness varies from two to 18 hours, although abdominal cramps, diarrhea, nausea, and vomiting usually occur about four hours after eating the poisoned food. In children, the incubation period may be shorter than in adults. Treatment is the same as for salmonella, though the symptoms of streptococcus poisoning are usually milder than in salmonella food poisoning.

Once again, sanitation and proper food cooking and storage is the key to prevention.

Vibrio parahaemolyticus

Vibrio parahaemolyticus, a close relative of the cholera organism, lives in sea water and is known to produce about half of the foodborne diseases in Japan, probably because raw fish is very popular there. Shipboard outbreaks on cruise liners have occurred when food has been inadvertently contaminated by sea water.

Evidence suggests that marinating raw fish in vinegar or lemon juice may decrease the activity of harmful organisms, but generally it is not a good idea to eat raw fish.

The organism's toxin is not known to be fatal, and treatment is symptomatic and supportive.

Worms

Various parasitic worms gain entrance to the human body through the medium of food. Some worms require an "intermediary host." For example, a dog acquires tapeworms from eating infected meat from another animal, then contaminates with his feces the playground of children who, thus, acquire the worms. Other worms are transmitted from man to man in food or water or are acquired from eating infected animal or fish meat.

Fish tapeworms

Fish tapeworms are often found in raw fish. When the fish are then eaten without cooking, the tapeworms can attach themselves to the small intestines of humans and grow to phenomenal lengths. Eating raw fish is not a good practice!

Trichinella spiralis

Trichinella spiralis is a minute worm that sometimes lies encysted in the muscles of the pig. When the live cysts are eaten by human beings, the worms invade the human's muscles. Trichinella are very widespread among pigs, and the practice of feeding raw garbage to hogs serves to perpetuate and spread the condition since untreated garbage is usually contaminated with trichinella spiralis larvae. Hog raisers should steam-sterilize all garbage before it is used for feeding purposes.

Unfortunately, only about seventy precent of the pork raised in this country is processed in plants that are under close sanitary inspection and a large part of our total supply of pork products may carry live parasites. It is important to realize that the cysts are almost invisible to the naked eye.

These parasites can be destroyed by heating the meat harboring them to at least 160°F or by freezing it at 5°F for twenty days or more. The condition can be prevented by the thorough cooking of all pork and pork products and avoidance of uncooked pork sausage meats. When cooking a pork roast, a thermometer inserted into the center of the thickest portion of the meat should read 185°F before the pork is eaten.

Symptoms occur after an incubation period of about one to two weeks, and they may include nausea, vomiting and diarrhea, muscular weakness, and stiffness or pain accompanied by fever. Swelling around the eye is common, and there is occasionally skin rash, headache, and visual disturbances. The great variety of symptoms, the variation in their intensity, and the irregularity in their course are characteristic of trichinosis. Medical attention is called for.

Food Poisoning Through Chemicals

Antimony

Antimony was often used as a binder between enamel and metal in old cooking utensils. Citric acid in fruit beverages may dissolve the binding in the worn enamel coating of large pans or other containers, thus releasing sufficient antimony to cause symptoms of poisoning. Treatment is symptomatic.

Arsenic

Arsenic is used in insecticides, ant poisons, weed killers, wallpaper, paint, ceramics, and glass. The possibility of accidental food contamination definitely exists. Additionally, recent medical literature contains a report of two women who were undergoing neurological examinations and were found to have elevated levels of arsenic. The arsenic was traced to the ingestion by these patients of health food supplements in tablet form prepared from kelp. The question is raised of possible adverse effects of long-continued daily ingestion of arsenic in this apparently readily absorbable form.

Symptomatology is entirely dependent on the amount ingested or inhaled. When massive amounts of arsenic are ingested, initial symptoms are violent gastroenteritis with vomiting and copious watery or bloody diarrhea and burning esophageal pain. There is a sweetish metallic taste with garlicky odor of breath and stools. Later the skin becomes cold and clammy. There is generalized weakness and the blood pressure falls. Convulsions and coma are the terminal signs and death is from circulatory failure. Inhalation of arsenic dusts may cause fatigue, difficulty in breathing, and a cough with a foamy sputum. Skin involvement may also occur. Immediate medical attention is needed.

Cadmium

If acid foods such as citrus fruit juices are placed in cadmium-plated utensils such as pitchers or refrigerator ice-trays, a sufficient amount of cadmium is dissolved to cause abdominal cramping, severe diarrhea, and vomiting within fifteen to thirty minutes after eating or drinking contaminated foods or beverages. Supportive and symptomatic treatment should be given.

Lead

Large doses would rarely be ingested except by those individuals who are "paint and putty eaters." However, contamination of food during preparation with the insecticide lead arsenate does occasionally occur as does contamination from the use of lead water pipes or lead-containing pottery. Nausea, vomiting, diarrhea, and cramps are early symptoms. Diagnosis and treatment require the attention of a physician.

Mercury

Compounds of mercury, especially in fish and shellfish, have caused widely publicized incidents of poisoning in human beings. Rivers have been carrying mercury into the oceans for millions of centuries. Mercury also enters the ocean from volcanoes. At present, about 10,000 tons of mercury flow into the sea each year, about one half of this is of natural origin, and the other half results from modern industrial activities developed within the past 200 years. It is interesting, therefore, to find out that tuna caught ninety years ago and preserved as a museum specimen, contains about the same level of mercury as canned tuna does today. With the exception of gross contamination such as occured in Minamata Bay, Japan, mercury poisoning by eating fish is unlikely.

Nature has its own way of coping with excess amounts of mercury, it has been discovered. Selenium, a trace element found in sea water, counteracts the toxic effects of methyl mercury. It has been shown that the selenium content of tuna runs parallel to the mercury content, thus preventing poisoning. Nature is, indeed, amazing!

Sodium fluoride

This insecticide is widely used to exterminate cockroaches from food establishments. Since it is a white powder, it can easily be mistaken for baking powder, soda, or flour. Illness follows within a few minutes to two hours after ingestion and is characterized by vomiting, diffuse abdominal pain, and diarrhea. Convulsions, paralysis of certain groups of muscles, hiccups, and contraction of the pupils may occur.

Initial home treatment should include milk, but definitive treatment with calcium should be given by a physician.

Tin and copper

Food poisoning has resulted from contamination of fruit punch with tin. The unusually high acid content of the punch can cause a chemical reaction with the lining of the container, resulting in gastrointestinal irritation. This can also occur if copper utensils are used. Recovery occurs in five to six hours. Therapy is symptomatic and supportive.

Zinc

Acid foods or liquids prepared or stored in galvanized zinc containers may dissolve sufficient zinc salts to produce severe vomiting, diarrhea, and prostration. Treatment is symptomatic.

Poisonous Plants and Seafood

Ergot

Ergot poisoning occurs from eating rye meal or rye bread prepared from rye diseased with ergot, a rust or fungus which contains a number of toxic alkaloids. Ergotism is rare in the United States, but outbreaks are still occasionally reported from eastern Europe.

Symptoms are drowsiness, headache, giddiness, painful cramps of the limbs, and itching of the skin. In severe cases, gangrene may occur, involving

Food Poisoning

the fingers and toes, and occasionally the ears and nose. Symptoms appear gradually, after several meals contained the diseased rye. Aside from elimination of the ergot-containing rye, treatment is symptomatic and supportive.

Mushrooms

There are several thousand species of mushrooms in the United States, but fortunately relatively few cause serious illness or death. There are three chief reasons for difficulties in distinguishing edible from poisonous forms. First, there are numerous species and the differences between them are rather subtle and require critical examination by someone specially trained for correct identification. Second, many species are variable in their characteristics, and poisonous qualities may also vary depending upon the season, habitat, and geographical area. Third, poisonous and edible forms may not only look alike to the nonspecialist but may grow together—even in the same fairy ring. In addition, the difficulties are magnified by variation in susceptibility among people.

The most poisonous of the mushrooms is Amanita phalloides; two or three of these white or yellow mushrooms are sufficient to cause illness and even death. More than half of those severely poisoned die. Findings include hypoglycemia which may be accompanied by convulsions, severe abdominal pain, intense thirst, nausea, retching, vomiting, and profuse watery stools. Illness ocurs within six to 15 hours after ingestion. Immediate attention is called for.

It should be noted that cooking will not destroy all the toxins in poisonous mushrooms and will not protect against the lethal effects in failure of proper identification. Nor is there any truth to the statements that a silver spoon or coin added to the pan in which mushrooms are cooked will darken if poisonous species are present. Also untrue is the notion that if the skin can be peeled from the cap of the mushroom and/or if the mushrooms fail to turn color when broken that they are nonpoisonous.

The common name *toadstool* (taken from *todessthul*—"death's stool"!) is often given to mushrooms that are poisonous, but there is no recognizable difference between the poisonous toadstool and the nonpoisonous mushroom. In fact, there is no simple rule of thumb for making this distinction. All such methods may work for a few species, but not for all. Beware of the mushroom "expert," for all too often he or she is more fortunate than expert.

Poisonous fish

The meat of approximately 300 species of fish causes poisoning when ingested. The commonest form of fish poisoning that occurs in the Caribbean area is called ciquatera. This is usually, but not always, caused by the meat of the moray eel or Sphyraena barracuda and is due to a toxin produced by certain algae which is ingested by the small plant-eating life of the reef which in turn are eaten by the fish. The grouper, snapper, and members of the wrasse family are other fish frequently involved.

Symptoms which appear thirty minutes after ingestion consist of nausea, vomiting, diarrhea, abdominal cramps, tingling, sweating, muscle weakness, and incoordination. Treatment is mainly symptomatic and supportive.

Potatoes

Solanine is found throughout the potato plant, with the highest concentrations in the unripened fruit. Misconceptions occur concerning the poisonous qualities of solanine, probably because of the harmless nature of the completely ripe potato. Solanine is, however, extremely toxic and small amounts can be deadly. Green and spoiled potatoes and potato sprouts have caused severe cases of poisoning. Never eat potatoes if they look spoiled or green below the skin, and always discard the sprouts.

Symptoms include headache, stomach pain, subnormal temperature, paralysis, dilated pupils, vomiting, diarrhea, shock, circulatory and respiratory depression, loss of sensation, and death. Medial attention is definitely called for.

Rhubarb

Rhubarb, commonly known for the edible leaf stalks, is quite poisonous if the leaf blades are eaten. The poisonous substance is possibly a soluble oxalate with an additional unknown toxin.

Symptoms include stomach pains, nausea, vomiting, weakness, difficulty of breathing, burning of mouth and throat, internal bleeding; coma and death can occur. Medical attention is required.

Scombroid

Scombroid poisoning is caused by a histaminelike subtance which produces in its human victims the symptoms of a severe allergy. Many reported cases of "fish sensitivity" are more correctly instances of scombroid poisoning following the ingestion of spoiled (through inadequate refrigeration or lack of freshness) mackerel-like fishes; even commercially canned tuna has occasionally been responsible.

The symptoms are similar to those of histamine poisoning. Within a few minutes after eating the toxic fish, which reportedly has a "peppery" or sharp taste, victims develop nausea and vomiting, flushing of the face, intense headache, epigastric pain, burning of the throat with difficulty in swallowing, thirst, and swelling of the lips. Soon they also develop massive red welts and intense itching. The symptoms usually subside within twelve hours. Treatment should

Food Poisoning

include administration of an antihistamine to relieve the victim's distress.

Shellfish

The consumption of mussels, clams, or crab has sporadically given rise to epidemics of poisoning in this country and abroad. In some instances the toxic effects are apparently caused by an allergic idiosyncrasy; in others, infection with salmonella organisms; and in many, poisoning due to toxic compounds which are especially concentrated in shellfish during the spawning season. In the latter, the symptoms resemble curare poisoning. It is characterized by paralysis of different groups of muscles, especially those of respiration. They vary from trembling about the lips to complete loss of power in the neck muscles. Nausea, vomiting, and diarrhea also occur. The illness develops within five to thirty minutes or longer after eating the poisoned food. The toxin is not destroyed by cooking. Medical attention is required.

Vicia faba bean

The plant from which this bean is taken is widely and commonly cultivated as an ornamental vine in various areas of southern United States. The beans are appearing in the markets both canned and frozen.

A type of poisoning known as "favism," which might be termed a food allergy but in reality is genetically related, is caused by this bean which is an important item in the diet of many Americans of Italian descent. Sensitization to the bean seems to be hereditary, since in certain families every member for generations has been reported to be severely affected. Susceptibility varies and a person long accustomed to eating the beans without ill effect may suffer a single, severe attack and experience none thereafter.

Favism produces a profound anemia, headache, dizziness, diarrhea, nausea and vomiting, abdominal pain, fever, and death in some cases. Inhalation of pollen from the flowers can cause headache and dizziness in two to three hours with more severe symptoms later. Medical attention is clearly called for. Transfusions may be necessary.

The beans may be eaten and the pollen inhaled without danger by those not carrying this genetic trait.

Water hemlock

The poisonous chemicals of water hemlock are found mostly in the rootstock and much less in the aboveground parts of the plant. The root is extremely poisonous, and one mouthful of root is sufficient to kill an adult. It is so often mistaken for wild parsnip or wild artichoke that deaths are frequent. Children have been poisoned by making peashooters and whistles from the hollow stems.

Symptoms occur within one to two hours after ingesting the poison and include diarrhea, violent convulsions and spasms, tremors, extreme stomach pain, dilated pupils, frothing at the mouth, delirium, and death. Immediate medical attention is required.

Antibiotic Residues

Antibiotic residues in foods pose a potential hazard to the health of human beings for several reasons. Persons sensitive to drugs such as penicillin and streptomycin may suffer adverse reactions from eating foods that carry residues of these antibiotics. Continued exposure to such drugs can contribute to the development of sensitization, which means that subsequent use of the antibiotics to treat an illness could cause adverse reactions. It is well established that bacteria that are continually exposed to antibiotics tend to develop resistance to these drugs. More restrictive use of antibiotics in food-producing animals will reduce the potential risk to man from residues in foods. We can hope that the Food and Drug Administration will take the necessary steps to prevent unauthorized and unsafe residues in foods.

Prevention of Food Poisoning

Control of food poisoning and infection depends mainly on proper methods of sanitation. Disease-producing bacteria in milk can be eliminated by sanitary processing, and most pathogens are destroyed in the pasteurization process. Water is subjected to a number of processes, such as chlorination, so that the real concern in controlling outbreaks today lies with food.

Many of the foods that cause poisoning receive no terminal sterilization, although some heat may be used in the cooking process. Staphylococcus bacteria—which are probably responsible for most food poisoning outbreaks—are easily destroyed in cooking, but they produce a heat-resistant toxin, so symptoms would be produced even without live bacteria. In addition, food cooked in public institutions and restaurants is exposed to many different handlers who are often unaware of, or indifferent to, the most elementary sanitary techniques. A stronger emphasis on the necessity of teaching sanitary techniques in secondary schools would be helpful in further enlightening people about the perils of food poisoning.

Most food poisonings are relatively mild. Often affected persons receive no medical treatment, and deaths are rare. Therefore, many outbreaks go unreported. This is unfortunate because the reporting of one outbreak may prevent others by making public institutions and restaurants more conscious of the dangers of inadequate sanitary conditions.

In all cases of food poisoning it is important to recognize the type, so recurrences can be prevented. Often there is no really specific treatment. Vomiting and diarrhea serve the useful purpose of eliminating poisons not already absorbed. Symptomatic treatment is usually all that is necessary.

Tips for Avoiding Food Poisoning

- Wash your hands before preparing food, after handling raw meats, and after blowing your nose or smoking. Keep fingernails clean.
- Use only clean clothing, aprons, towels, and equipment.
- Avoid using hands to mix foods and keep hands away from mouth, nose, and hair.
- A person with a skin infection or infectious disease should not prepare food. Avoid coughing or sneezing over foods.
- Refrigerate all perishables soon after purchase and refrigerate leftovers promptly, using shallow pans — they will cool faster. And don't leave the stuffing in meat of fowl.
- Keep hot foods at 150°F or higher and cold foods at 40-45°F or lower. Bacteria grow rapidly at in-between temperatures.
- Freezing cannot be relied on to sterilize food, and frozen foods, once thawed, should be regarded as particularly perishable products.
- Do not remove cold foods from the refrigerator more than one-half hour before serving. Add dressings to salads just before serving.
- Whenever there is any reason to doubt the freshness or wholesomeness of a food, it should never be consumed and should be disposed of in such a fashion that small children and domestic animals cannot reach and eat it.
- When eating out, beware of buffets where food may be displayed for hours.
- Report to your physician or local health authority any case of food poisoning so that other cases may be prevented.

Many of the above rules are especially important when preparing food for or attending picnics or large group dinners.

Appendix I—Recipes

Main Meals Which Convert to Great Lunchbox Ideas

As we spoke to the many people with whom we consulted during the course of writing this book, it became apparent that lunchtime presents a real problem. Many of us are away from home for this meal and either have to take our lunches with us or we are at the mercy of the school or office cafeteria, vending machines, or some other fast food service facility. The luncheon recipes that follow are, therefore, all geared to being prepared ahead of time; packed; stored without reheating or refrigeration for at least half a day. A wide-mouth hot/cold thermos is a must, however.

Cold cuts, cheese, and peanut butter may well be purchased especially for lunch-making, but a bit more variety can be introduced if dinner leftovers are also used. A little imagination is often all that is needed. To get you started, we have included a few menus and recipes for main meals and the adaptations necessary to turn your leftovers into lunches "with a difference."

You will notice that all of the following meal plans are meatless. Most families are quite familiar with a variety of meat dishes, but vegetables are usually looked upon merely as supporting members of the cast, with meat being the star of the meal. Considering today's high meat prices, it is time for vegetables to assume a more important role.

Many cultures obtain the majority of their protein from grains. For example, in the Asian countries, only about 14 percent of the protein consumed daily is from animals (mainly milk), compared to 68 percent in the United States. There are, thus, many delicious meatless recipes available to you. We hope that the following samples will start you on the road of discovery.

The recipes have been planned to maximize the amount of usable protein, and to use ingredients readily available. And even if you aren't familiar with some of the foods, we think you'll find these dishes very easy to prepare. You'll be pleasantly surprised to find just how little time and effort are involved.

If you'd like to learn more about meeting your nutrient requirements when planning meatless meals, read the chapter on Vegetarianism—Fad or a Different Way?

The Commonsense Guide to Good Eating

Want to share your special recipes with others? Then why not send them to us for possible inclusion in a later book. Please make sure that you include your name and address so that we can give you proper recognition for your contribution.

MEAL PLANS

Menu No.	Dinner Menu	Lunchbox Adaptation
I	Barley casserole* Lima Beans with mushrooms* Spiced cornbread*	Vegetable-barley soup* Cornbread
II	Meatless loaf* Glazed carrots Raw spinach-mushroom salad with Italian dressing	Loaf sandwich* Raw carrot sticks
III	Broiled eggplant sandwich* Tabbouleh salad*	Pocket sandwich* Cheese cubes
IV	Cheese-onion pie* Marinated broccoli* Sauteed apples	Cheese-onion pie Broccoli soup* Peanut butter apple*
V	Mujaddarah* Riata* Arab bread*	Lentil-yogurt salad* Bread sticks
VI	Soybean chili* Cheese tortillas* Shredded lettuce and tomatoes	Leftover chili Tortilla chips*

Drinks	Miscellaneous
Acerola cocktail* Carob delight* Orange shake*	Marge's never-fail bread* Flavored fruit yogurt* Bean sprouts*

*Recipes for starred items included.

Appendix I—Recipes

MENU NO. 1

Barley Casserole
makes 6 servings

Ingredients	Exchange List
1½ cups uncooked barley	12 Bread
3½ cups water (vegetable broth would give more flavor)	Free Food
1 onion, chopped	1 Grp. B Vegetable
½ green pepper, chopped	Grp. A Vegetable
1 tomato chopped	
Salt and pepper to taste	Free Food
1 tbsp. oil	3 Fat
¼ tsp. oregano, basil, or Italian seasoning	Free Food
1 cup grated cheese	4 Meat

1. Preheat oven to 375° F.
2. Combine all ingredients *except* cheese in a covered baking dish. Place in oven.
3. After 45 minutes, remove from oven, stir in cheese, and mix thoroughly. Cover and bake for another 15 minutes.
4. If desired, sprinkle a little extra cheese on top and bake, uncovered, an additional 5 minutes or until cheese melts.

Each serving equals: 2 Bread, ½ Fat, and ½ Meat exchanges. (The negligible amount of Group B Vegetable need not be counted.)

Lima Beans with Mushrooms
makes 6 servings

Ingredients	Exchange List
3 cups cooked lima beans	6 Bread
1 cup mushroom slices or pieces, cooked or raw	Grp. A Vegetable
Hot sauce of choice	Free Food

1. Put all ingredients in pan, adding just enough other liquid to keep contents from burning. Cover and cook over low heat until hot.

Each serving equals: 1 Bread exchange.

The Commonsense Guide to Good Eating

Spiced Cornbread

To your favorite cornbread recipe, add chopped onions and/or chili powder before baking. Each 1½ inch cube of cornbread equals 1 Bread exchange.

Vegetable-Barley Soup

Combine leftover Barley Casserole and Lima Beans with Mushrooms with enough broth, bouillon, or water to make soup. Add any other interesting leftovers that you may have. Season to taste and heat thoroughly. You'll want to keep an eye on this as it thickens rather rapidly. You may need to add additional liquid. Each cup of soup equals 1 Bread exchange.

MENU NO. II

Meatless Loaf
about 6 servings

Ingredients	Exchange List
¼ cup oil	12 Fat
1 cup onions, chopped	2 Grp. B Vegetables
1 cup any combination of: diced celery, green pepper, fresh parsley, drained tomatoes, carrots, squash, beans, olives, etc.	Check lists for ingredients used
1 cup nuts of choice, finely chopped (you'll find your blender very handy for this job) *or* 1 cup chunky style peanut butter	
1 cup *cooked* brown or white rice*	2 Bread
⅓ cup bread crumbs (whole wheat, rye, pumpernickle, etc.) good way to use up stale bread	2 Bread
1 cup grated cheese of choice	4 Meat
2 eggs, beaten	2 Meat
¼ tsp. pepper	Free Food

1. Preheat oven to 350° F.
2. Cook onions and any other vegetables used in the oil until just limp.
3. Combine fried vegetables and all remaining ingredients. Mix well. Add a

Appendix I—Recipes

small amount of liquid (milk, broth, water) if mixture seems too dry. This may be necessary especially when using peanut butter.
4. Place in greased loaf pan and bake for about 40 minutes. One of the new non-stick pans may prove useful if you plan to unmold the loaf before serving.

*Why not cook up a large batch of rice at one time. Freeze extra amounts in small containers for later use. You may also want to try cooking rice in meat or vegetable stock rather than in plain water.

Loaf Sandwich

Not much to do here, thanks to last night's leftovers. Spread bread or roll of choice with mustard and/or ketchup. Add lettuce or drained bean sprouts and a slice of chilled Meatless Loaf, and you're finished.

MENU NO. III

Broiled Eggplant Sandwich
Variable

Even people who don't usually care for for eggplant seem to like this dish.

Ingredients	Exchange List
Eggplant	Grp. A Vegetable
Oil	1 Fat for ea. tsp.
Slices of thick dark bread	1 Bread per slice
Garlic butter	see Fat list
Bean sprouts (optional)	Grp. A Vegetable
Mozzarella or other cheese, sliced	1 Meat per oz.
Salt and pepper	Free Food

1. If desired, partially peel the raw eggplant by removing lengthwise strips of peeling to give eggplant a striped effect. Leaving strips of peeling will help keep the eggplant from falling apart when cooking. Now, slice the eggplant horizontally into 3/4 inch slices.
2. Fry eggplant slices in hot oil until brown on both sides and tender throughout. (The eggplant will absorb a fair amount of oil cooked this way. An alternative method of cooking is to brush the eggplant slices with oil and

then broil them. Cooked this way, much less oil need be used.) Drain the slices on a paper towel.
3. Spread the bread slices with the garlic butter (toast bread first if crispness is desired). Top with bean sprouts and slices of cooked eggplant. Add salt and pepper to taste. Arrange cheese slices on top of eggplant. Put in oven and broil until cheese is melted.

Tabbouleh Salad
serves 8

This is one of our favorite Lebanese dishes. We think your whole family will love it.

Ingredients	Exchange List
1 cup raw cracked wheat (bulgur)	8 Bread
Water	Free Food
1 cup finely chopped onions	2 Group B Vegetable
1 cup finely chopped fresh parsley (fresh parsley really makes a taste difference)	Grp. A Vegetable
1 cup chopped fresh tomatoes	
¼ cup dried, crushed mint (or ½ cup fresh, finely chopped mint)	Free Food
⅓ cup lemon juice	
⅓ cup olive oil	12 Fat
Salt and pepper to taste	

1. Cover the cracked wheat with water and set aside for one hour to allow wheat to soften. Then drain water off cracked wheat, pressing out any excess water with your hands.
2. Combine all remaining ingredients; add drained cracked wheat. Toss well and chill.

Each serving equals: 1 Bread and 1½ Fat exchanges. The amount of Group B Vegetables is too minimal to worry about.

Pocket Sandwich

The typical bread of Arab countries is a flat, round loaf which is only slightly leavened. As the bread cooks in the oven, it puffs up but falls as it cools. A pocket is thus formed which can be filled with whatever your imagination dictates.

This bread is found in other parts of the world as well, being known by many different names — khubz, Arab bread, flat bread, pocket bread, pita, bible bread,

Appendix I—Recipes

etc. It comes made with either white or whole wheat flour. You're more likely to find this delicious bread in a specialty store rather than at the local supermarket—or you can make it yourself.

1. Using your favorite yeast bread recipe or a box of hot roll mix, prepare according to directions, letting dough rise once. Then punch down and shape it into three or more balls (the number of balls depends upon how much dough you have and how large you want the finished products to be). Let balls rise, covered, for about one hour. Once again, punch down dough and then roll out each dough ball to about five inches in diameter (or whatever size you prefer). Cover dough circles and wait about one more hour.
2. Place cookie sheet in oven on rack approximately five to six inches away from broiler heat. Turn broiler on high and heat oven and cookie sheet for about five minutes before adding dough. Now, partially pull the rack out and place two or three (depending on their size) dough circles on the cookie sheet. Return the rack to its original position, leave oven door ajar, and broil dough circles for about 2 minutes or until light brown. Turn dough and broil another couple of minutes.
3. Remove bread from oven and place in a covered pan. Cool bread by storing it warm and allowing the steam to release of its own accord. Otherwise, bread will be hard. Cook remaining dough circles.

This bread freezes well and can be reheated readily. To make a pocket sandwich using last night's leftovers, simply place the Tabbouleh in a wide-mouth thermos. At lunch time, spoon the Tabbouleh into the flat Arab bread which has been cut in half (so that you can get at the pocket) and enjoy!

MENU NO. IV

Cheese-Onion Pie
serves 6

Ingredients	Exchange List
1 9-inch pie pastry	9 Bread
2 tbsp. oil or butter	6 Fat
2 med. onions, chopped	2 Grp. B Vegetables
½ lb. cheese, cubed or grated	8 Meat
3 eggs	3 Meat
⅛ tsp. nutmeg	Free Food
1 sm. can evaporated milk (unsweetened)	1 Milk per 4 ozs.

1. Line a 9-inch pie plate with pastry. (If you're making your own, try using

whole wheat pastry flour rather than white all purpose flour—you might find it a pleasant change.) Prick pastry with fork to prevent it from puffing when cooking. Bake in 400°F oven for about 8 minutes. Remove from oven and set aside.
2. Fry onions in butter or oil until tender and golden. Spread cooked onions over bottom of pastry. Sprinkle cheese on top of onions.
3. Combine eggs, nutmeg, and a small amount of the canned milk. Pour over onions and cheese in pie crust. Add as much more of the canned milk as the pie will hold without overflowing.
4. Bake in a preheated 350°F oven for 35 minutes or until custard is set.

Good hot or cold. Each serving equals: 1½ Bread, 1 Fat, and approximately 2 Meat exchanges. There is not enough Group B Vegetable or Milk to worry about.

If making your own pastry for the cheese-onion pie, you can make an individual-size pie for tomorrow's lunch simply by lining one or more muffin tin spaces with dough and then proceeding as above. You can also make a small piecrust by rolling out a refrigerator biscuit to fit the muffin space.

Marinated Broccoli
Variable

Ingredients	Exchange List
Raw broccoli, cleaned and cut into bite-size pieces	Grp. A Vegetable
1 cup vinegar	Free Food
1 tbsp. sugar	1 Bread
1 tbsp. dill weed	
1 tsp. pepper	Free Food
1 tsp. garlic salt	
1½ cups vegetable oil	59 Fat

Combine all ingredients and let marinate, preferably overnight.

Appendix I—Recipes

Broccoli Soup
Variable

Ingredients	Exchange List
Broccoli, fresh, frozen, or marinated from last night's leftovers	Grp. A Vegetable
Tomatoes, squash, etc.—any vegetables you have around	See Lists
Vegetable broth	} Free Food
Garlic powder	
Grated cheese	See Meat List

Cut broccoli into bite-size pieces and add to vegetable broth; if using plain water, flavor it with salt and pepper and a bit of thyme. Add any other vegetables that you want. Actually the soup requires no other and is delicious plain. Add a dash of garlic powder. Cook until vegetables are tender. Usually served with grated cheese on top, but you may want to omit this when serving the soup with the cheese-onion pie.

Peanut Butter Apple
serves 1

Ingredients	Exchange List
1 apple, cored	1 Fruit
2 tbsp. peanut butter	1 Meat

Fill cored apple with peanut butter for a simple, surprisingly delicious treat!

MENU NO. V

Mujaddarah
serves 8

A delicious Lebanese dish. Recipes often call for rice rather than cracked wheat, but we think this recipe to be even tastier.

Ingredients	Exchange List
1 cup uncooked lentils	4 Bread
1 cup raw cracked wheat (bulgur)	8 Bread

The Commonsense Guide to Good Eating

Ingredients	Exchange List
3 ¾ cups vegetable broth, bouillon, or water (if plain water is used, flavor it with salt, pepper and a dash of garlic powder)	Free Food
2 medium-sized onions, sliced lengthwise	2 Grp. B Vegetables
¼ cup oil	12 Fat
8 tomatoes, cut into small pieces	Grp. A Vegetables
½ cup chopped fresh parsley	Free Food
6 scallions, thinly sliced	1 Grp. B Vegetable
Juice from 1 large lemon	Free Food

1. Bring liquid to a boil; add lentils and cracked wheat. Reduce heat to low, cover pan, and cook until liquid is absorbed—about 15 minutes.
2. While lentils and cracked wheat are cooking, cook the onions in the olive oil over medium heat until the onions are limp.
3. Combine the tomatoes, parsley, scallions, and lemon juice.
4. When the lentils and cracked wheat are cooked and the onions are limp, combine them.
5. Now for the surprise! The hot lentil-cracked wheat-onion mixture is served *over* the tomato-parsley salad!

Each serving equals: 1½ Bread, 1½ Fat, and negligible Group B Vegetable exchanges.

Riata
Variable

Ingredients	Exchange List
Unpeeled, thinly sliced (or peeled chunks) cucumber	Grp. A Vegetable
Chopped green peppers	
Yogurt thinned with buttermilk	½ Milk per ½ cup
Dill weed, lemon pepper, seasoned salt to taste	Free Food

1. Combine all ingredients and chill.

Chopped tomatoes make a good addition to this dish when it isn't to be served with another dish having tomatoes as a main ingredient.

Lentil-Yogurt Salad

Combine leftover Mujaddarah and Riata. Chill. Makes a delicious cold salad for tomorrow's lunch or an excellent filling for a Pocket Sandwich.

Appendix I—Recipes

Arab Bread

See Pocket Sandwich.

MENU NO. VI

Soybean Chili
serves 6

Try using your favorite recipe for chili (with or without meat) but substitute cooked soybeans for the usual kidney or other beans. Or try the following recipe.

Ingredients	Exchange List
2 tbsp. oil	6 Fat
1 med. onion, chopped	1 Grp. B Vegetable
1 green pepper, cut in strips	Grp. A Vegetable
4 cups (2 cans) cooked soybeans	3 Meat
4 cups (2 cans) tomatoes	Grp. A Vegetable
2 tbsp. chopped parsley	
1 tbsp. chili powder	
1 tsp. ground cumin seed	Free Food
½ tsp. garlic powder	
1 tbsp. jalapeno chili sauce (optional—very hot)	
1 cup yogurt	1 Milk

1. Cook onion and green pepper in oil until just limp.
2. Add all remaining ingredients *except* yogurt. Cook over low heat (cover pan) for about 1 hour, stirring occasionally.
3. Serve with a "dollop" of plain yogurt on top.

Each serving equals: 1 Fat, ½ Meat, and negligible Group B Vegetable and Milk exchanges.

Green soybeans are a dependable source of a number of minerals and vitamins including calcium, phosphorus, iron, vitamin A, thiamin, and riboflavin. However, a considerable portion of the vitamin A is lost during drying. Dry soybeans contain 1½ times as much protein (including all the essential amino acids) as other dry beans and 11 times as much fat; the fat is high in polyunsaturated fatty acids.

Cheese Tortillas
Variable

Ingredients	Exchange List
Tortillas	1 Bread each
Cheese	1 Meat per oz.
Oil	1 Fat per tsp.

Fold tortillas in half. Fill with grated or sliced cheese. Bake at 350°F until cheese is melted. If you like your tortillas crispier than this, fry or brush with oil and bake them before adding the cheese.

Tortilla Chips

Brush both sides of tortilla with oil. Cut into strips or wedges. Place on cookie sheet and sprinkle lightly with onion salt or other seasoning of choice. Bake in 400°F oven until light brown—about 10 minutes. Cool before storing in an airtight container.

DRINKS

Acerola Cocktail

Acerola is a fruit related to the cherry that grows in the West Indies. A half cup of acerola juice contains almost thirty times the amount of vitamin C as does the same amount of orange juice! Acerola powder can be found usually in a health food store. Mix it with water or milk for a new taste treat.

Carob Delight
serves 1

Carob powder, obtained from the beans of the carob tree, is an excellent substitute for chocolate. Not only is it much lower in calories than chocolate or cocoa, it contains almost no fat, is a relatively good source of protein, and contains none of the stimulants found in chocolate. (Incidentally, in substituting carob powder for chocolate, 3 tablespoons of carob plus 2 tablespoons of water or milk equals 1 square of chocolate.)

Ingredients	Exchange List
1 cup milk	1 Milk
1½ tsp. carob powder	Negligible Fat
⅛ tsp. vanilla	Free Food
1 tsp. sugar, honey or blackstrap molasses,	Negligible
or ½ banana	1 Fruit
For a change of pace sometime, try adding 1 tsp. instant coffee; use decaffinated coffee if you're trying to avoid caffeine.	Free Food

Blend well. Serve hot or cold. When this mixture is put in a blender, it gets quite foamy. When heated, it boils over easily, so be carefeul. (If neither using a blender or the instant type of carob powder, you may want to dissolve the carob powder in a bit of hot water to make it blend more readily.)

Orange Shake
serves 1

Ingredients	Exchange List
1 cup chilled orange juice	2 Fruit
¼ cup powdered milk	1 Milk
1 tsp. sugar	Neglibile
⅛ tsp. vanilla	} Free Food
Crushed ice	

Blend well.

MISCELLANEOUS

Marge's Never-Fail Bread
2 loaves

Sometimes an interesting bread makes all the difference in the world when

The Commonsense Guide to Good Eating

planning a meal. Following is a basic recipe to get you started that a friend of ours was kind enough to share. Experiment with different flours and seasonings.

Ingredients	Exchange List
1 cup warm water 1 package dry yeast 1 cup warm water 3 tbsp. sugar 1 tbsp. salt ¼ cup salad oil	Negligible

1. Combine ingredients in the above order. Stir well.
2. Add 2 cups flour. Stir. Add 2 more cups flour and stir. Knead a bit and add flour (about 1 cup) so you can handle without getting too stuck in the mixture. Do not add more than is necessary. Let rise in bowl (grease top with oil and cover bowl with wax paper or clean towel) until about double in size.
3. Then knead for 3-5 minutes or less depending on your mood and how big a hurry you are in. Divide into 2 loaves. Place in well-buttered bread pans. Rub lightly with oil. Let rise until about double in bulk again.
4. Bake at 350°F for 30 minutes. Turn out on wire rack immediately. This bread is almost impossible to ruin!

Flavored Fruit Yogurt
serves 1

Ingredients	Exchange List
1 cup plain yogurt	1 Milk
1 tbsp. frozen orange juice concentrate	Negligible Fruit
2 tbsp. raisins or other chopped dried fruit of choice	1 Fruit
1 tbsp. chopped nuts of choice	1 Fat

Mix well. Keep chilled.

Bean Sprouts

If you've never tried sprouting beans or seeds, you ought to give it a try. It is simple, fun, and economical. Almost all whole seeds, grains, and dried beans will sprout, but make sure that you never eat potato sprouts as they are poisonous. Sprouts will reach their optimum length in two to five days, depending on the seed or bean used.

Appendix I—Recipes

The following example uses soybeans which increase in volume about six times as they sprout. That is, $1/3$ cup of dry beans will yield about 2 cups of sprouts.
1. A clean clay flowerpot or milk carton makes a suitable container for sprouting. Cover the hole in the flowerpot with cheesecloth to hold beans in while allowing water to drain out freely, or punch small holes in the sides and bottom of the milk carton.
2. Soak the soybeans overnight in about three times as much water as beans. Rinse the soaked beans well and place in the prepared container.
3. Set the container in a cool place. Rinse the beans with cool water four or five times a day. It is important that all the water drains out to prevent growth of mold. If any beans become moldy , throw them out.
4. The sprouts will be 2 to 3 inches in 3 to 5 days, but may be eaten before that if desired. Soybean sprouts may be stored for 3 to 5 days in a tightly sealed jar or plastic bag in the refrigerator.

Appendix II—
Vitamins and Minerals

Vitamins

Vitamins are organic compounds that are necessary in small amounts for normal growth, maintenance of health, and reproduction. The action of vitamins is not unlike that of trace elements, in that the presence or absence of very small amounts of them in food can mean the difference between normal and abnormal functioning of the body.

Traditionally, vitamins are divided into two groups on the basis of their solubility: fat-soluble vitamins and water-soluble vitamins. Though the four fat-soluble vitamins (A, D, E, K) have quite different chemical properties, they have a few general distinctive similarities that distinguish them from the water-soluble vitamins.

1. They are more stable in heat than the water-soluble vitamins and are less likely to be lost in the cooking and processing of foods.

2. Fat-soluble vitamins are absorbed from the intestine along with fats and lipids in foods, so that anything that interferes with fat absorption results in lowered utilization of these vitamins. This is not a problem for water-soluble vitamins.

3. Because fat-soluble vitamins are not soluble in water, they are not excreted in the urine. Instead they are stored in the body, mainly in the liver, to a considerable extent. Hence deficiency symptoms may be slow in developing and low-grade shortages may be hard to detect. In contrast, water-soluble vitamins are not stored in the body in appreciable quantities, and a constant dietary supply of these vitamins is desirable to avoid their depletion.

4. Because fat-soluble vitamins can be stored in the body, toxicity—a poisonous state—may develop if too great an amount is ingested, for the excess cannot be excreted in the urine. Excesses of the water-soluble vitamins, however, are usually excreted in the urine and, hence, toxicity does not often occur. This does not mean that excessive amounts of these vitamins can be

taken without fear of harm, as you will see when you read about ascorbic acid (Vitamin C).

The Fat-Soluble Vitamins

Vitamin A
Function: Vitamin A is essential for growth, vision in dimly lighted areas, tooth development, and maintenance of the quality of the skin.

Excess: Hypervitaminosis A, caused by long-term high doses of this vitamin, has resulted in serious toxic (poisonous) states, especially in young children. Symptoms include: excessive irritability, swellings over the long bones, dry and itching skin, headaches, nausea, vomiting, diarrhea, and enlargement of the liver and spleen. Excessive intake can result in unlocalized intracranial pressure, often referred to as "pseudotumor cerebri syndrome." A great excess of this vitamin can lead to decalcification of bones with consequent fragility.

Unfortunately, people sometimes self-administer large amounts of this vitamin to themselves or their children in the hopes of improving their vision, preventing colds, or clearing up skin conditions. These abuses, with their serious consequences, contributed to the Food and Drug Administration's proposal to restrict the over-the-counter sale of high-dosage preparations. Regular ingestion of more than 2000 retinol equivalents (6700 IU) of preformed vitamin A above that already in the diet should be carefully monitored by a physician.

Deficiency: As the body stores large amounts of this vitamin, a person's diet would have to be deficient in liver, dairy products, and fresh vegetables for a long time before any clinical effects would be seen. Unfortunately, this seems to be the case for some of our population. Long-term insufficiency can result in stunted growth; roughness of skin; night blindness; damage to the linings of the mouth, throat, nose; and respiratory passages; as well as abnormalities in the enamel-forming cells of the teeth.

In animals, a vitamin A deficiency has serious effects in pregnancy and is a cause of infertility and congenital deformities.

Food sources: The chief sources of preformed vitamin A (retinol) are fish-liver oils, liver, kidney, egg yolk, butter, whole milk, cheese made from whole milk, deep yellow and dark green leafy vegetables, and tomatoes. Both vitamins A and D are often added to products such as ready-to-eat cereals, flavoring agents for milk, and "instant" meals.

Carotenes of plant origin are readily converted into vitamin A by the liver, where it is stored and from which it is released as needed by the tissues. In the prolonged ingestion of carotene foods (carrots, yellow squash, sweet

Appendix II—Vitamins and Minerals

potatoes, spinach, oranges, yellow corn and beans, egg yolks, butter, kale, apple juice, pumpkins, turnips, parsnips, rutabagas, and papaya) and in diabetes, hypothyroidism, and disorders of the liver, the conversion of carotene may be disturbed and it may appear in unusual amounts in the blood, producing carotenemia, an innocuous condition in which the skin—particularly the soles and the palms—shows a yellow discoloration. The eyes, however, are not involved. The possibility of symptomatic vitamin A intoxication from a diet high in carotenoids would be most unlikely. Lycopenemia, a condition similar to carotenemia except the skin is more highly tinted a deep orange-yellow, is due to high levels of lycopene in the liver and blood from excessive ingestion of tomato juice, rarely from beets, rose hips, (berries left on rose bushes), and reddish foods such as chili.

RDA: Males, 11-51+ years: 1000 RE (5000 IU). Females, 11-51+ years: 800 RE (4000 IU). See Table 1 for needs of infants, children, pregnant and nursing women.

Until recently, vitamin A activity in foods has been expressed as international units (IU). However, because of the poorer utilization of dietary provitamins (substances such as carotenes which are capable of being converted into a vitamin) as compared to preformed vitamin A (retinol), the expression of the total vitamin A activity of a diet as IU has had to be qualified by indicating the percentages of the activity coming from retinol and coming from provitamins. Needless to say, this causes a degree of confusion in estimating vitamin A activity. Until "retinol equivalents" becomes standard labeling, the Food and Nutrition Board of the National Academy of Sciences has recommended that dietary allowances for vitamin A be given both as retinol equivalents and as international units.

In the United States, the usual foods available to the consumer are estimated to provide about half of the total vitamin A activity as retinol and half as provitamin A carotenoids. By definition, one retinol equivalent is equal to 1 mcg of retinol, or 6 mcg of β-carotene, or 12 mcg of other provitamin A carotenoids. In terms of international units, one retinol equivalent is equal to 3.33 IU of retinol or 10 IU of β-carotene.

Vitamin D

Function: Vitamin D, the sunshine vitamin, is not only necessary to promote bone and tooth growth, but it also improves the body's utilization of calcium and phosphorus.

Excess: Toxicity (poisoning) occurs much easier with vitamin D than vitamin A. Abnormally high levels of calcium appear in the blood and symptoms may include: loss of appetite, vomiting, diarrhea, weakness, intense thirst, weight loss, headache, drowsiness, kidney damage, and retarded growth.

Amounts of vitamin D above 2000 IU per day for prolonged periods are dangerous to both infants and adults.

The most common cause of hypervitaminosis D is the new parent who gives the child extra vitamins in the hopes of "insuring" his or her development. Adults sometimes fall prey to the toxic effects of this vitamin when they have taken massive doses for arthritis or other conditions. One can easily see why the Food and Drug Administration feels the need to restrict the availability of high-dosage preparations and to consider limiting the enrichment of foods other than milk.

Deficiency: Despite the paucity of this vitamin in most natural foods, the practice of fortifying or enriching foods with vitamin D leaves little likelihood of a deficiency occuring—if one drinks fortified milk. Unfortunately, however, there still remains a considerable amount of unfortified milk.

When a deficiency does occur, it results in inadequate intestinal absorption of calcium and phosphorous and in increased loss of these minerals in the urine and feces. This results in demineralization of the bone. In adults, this causes a softening of the bone called osteomalacia. In actively growing children, the result is rickets, a skeletal malformtion.

Food sources: Only a few foods provide this vitamin. The only rich source are the liver oils of fish. Unfortified milk and meat contain only a negligible amount, while enriched cereals, vegetables, and fruit contain no vitamin D at all. Thus, it is easy to see why the practice of fortifying milk began. Sunshine helps the body to manufacture its own store of this vitamin from the action of ultraviolet light on sterols in the skin.

RDA: Males and females, 11-22 years: 400 IU. See Table 1 for requirements for others.

Vitamin E

Function: Vitamin E has been called the sex vitamin because vitamin E deficiency in rats can lead to sterility in males and spontaneous abortion in females. There is no convincing evidence that deficiencies of this vitamin in man have anything to do with reproductive functions, or that extra amounts of this vitamin improve one's sexual interest or abilities—sad but true!

Now, for what it can do. Vitamin E, because of its antioxidant properties, helps prevent cell membrane damage from certain naturally occuring body chemicals and protects both vitamin A and carotene—which can be converted to vitamin A—from destruction within the body.

Excess: So far, there is no evidence that high doses of this vitamin are poisonous, which is in marked contrast to the other fat-soluble vitamins.

Deficiency: Vitamin E is found in most foods and, therefore, dietary deficiency is unlikely. However, some infants are born with an inadequate reserve of this vitamin, resulting in anemia.

Appendix II—Vitamins and Minerals

Food sources: The richest sources are fats of vegetable origin (salad oils), particularly those derived from corn, soya bean, peanut, coconut, or cottonseed. Cereal products and eggs are the next best source.

RDA: Males, 11-14 years: 12 IU; 15-51+ years: 15 IU. Females, 11-51+ years: 12 IU. See Table 1 for requirements for others.

Available evidence indicates that, in the United States, the vitamin E content of diets varies widely, depending primarily on the amount and types of fat consumed (that is, animal versus vegetable fat) and the proportions in which they are consumed. Two reports based on analysis of foods as consumed indicated daily intakes of vitamin E from adult diets ranging from 2.6 to 15.4 mg, with an average of 7.4 mg (11 IU) in one case, and from 4.4 to 12.7 mg, with an average of 9.0 mg (13.4 IU) in the other.

Vitamin K

Function: Vitamin K is necessary for the formation in the liver of a substance called prothrombin, which is required for the normal clotting of blood.

Excess: Vitamin K_3, a synthetic compound, has been shown to produce toxicity in rats and human infants. Consequently, the Food and Drug Administration ordered the removal of this synthetic vitamin from all food supplements. The natural forms of K_1 and K_2 have not caused toxicity even when given in large amounts.

Deficiency: Dietary deficiency in adults has never been clearly demonstrated. Any condition that impairs fat absorption may, however, result in a vitamin K deficiency, thus slowing blood clotting time. It was once felt that bleeding in the newborn was due solely to the lack of vitamin K, but recent evidence points to deficiencies in other clotting factors.

Food sources: Excellent sources include: all green leafy vegetables, especially lettuce, spinach, and kale. Liver, egg yolk, soybean oil, cauliflower, and cabbage are also good sources.

RDA: Adequate information is not yet available about the amount of vitamin K the body requires. It is estimated that adults require about 50 mcg daily. Apparently, bacteria in the intestine provide considerable amounts of this vitamin for most people. However, when bacterial growth is suppressed by lengthy antibiotic therapy, vitamin K must be supplied.

The Water-Soluble Vitamins

Ascorbic acid (vitamin C)

Function: Ascorbic acid is necessary for the proper formation of substances that cement cells together such as capillaries, bone, teeth and connective tissue. This vitamin is also involved in protecting the body against infections, but recent claims that very large intakes of vitamin C can protect against the common cold are without good scientific evidence. There is some indication that this vitamin may reduce the cold sufferer's general feeling of malaise, but in view of the early evidence suggesting long-term serious complications, you would be better off to rely on simple symptomatic and supportive therapy.

Excess: The symptom noted most frequently is diarrhea. Recent studies have indicated that kidney problems may also arise. In experiments done on animals, the fetus was adversely affected by large doses of this vitamin. Also of concern is a recently published report suggesting that high doses of vitamin C (0.5 gm or more) may destroy substantial amounts of vitamin B_{12}; this would be of particular concern to pure vegetarians as they already have problems obtaining adequate amounts of vitamin B_{12} in their diet.

Deficiency: The most well-known effect of a serious and prolonged vitamin C deficiency is the development of scurvy, a disease which claimed the lives of many in the past but which is seldom seen today. There is some storing of this vitamin through tissue saturation, so unless your diet is really low in vegetables and fruits for a long period, a deficiency is unlikely to occur. Nonetheless, the recent United States Health and Nutrition Survey found clinical signs of vitamin C deficiency in a fraction of most age groups, regardless of sex or race.

Food sources: Vitamin C has a more limited food distribution than the other important water-soluble vitamins; we must depend almost entirely on fruits and vegetables. Citrus fruits, strawberries, cantaloupe, green leafy vegetables, peppers, broccoli, and cauliflower all are rich sources of vitamin C. Potatoes, though containing much smaller amounts of this vitamin, are an important food source because of the quantities of potatoes consumed.

Exposure to air as well as heat causes destruction of this very important vitamin. Therefore, buy fruits and vegetables in small quantities so that they are used promptly; do not let them stand in water or be exposed to air for long periods before eating or cooking them.

RDA: Males and females, 11-51+ years: 45 mg. See Table 1 for requirements for others.

There is some evidence that certain conditions of stress and drug therapy may call for increased amounts of vitamin C.

Biotin

Function: Biotin is important in the synthesis of fatty acids and the production of energy and in the formation of several amino acids.

Excess: No known effects.

Deficiency: The ingestion of eight to ten raw eggs a day by a person with a biotin-low diet can produce skin changes, loss of appetite, low-grade anemia, depression, and muscle pain. This is because raw egg white contains

Appendix II—Vitamins and Minerals

a protein called avidin which combines with biotin in the intestinal tract and keeps the biotin from being absorbed. The occassional eating of raw eggs, as in eggnog, will not provide enough avidin to produce a biotin deficiency.

Food sources: In addition to its availability through food supplies, microorganisms in the intestinal tract can synthesize this vitamin and, thus, there is little likelihood of a deficiency. Liver, kidney, and yeast extract are good sources. Some vegetables, nuts, and chocolate are fair sources.

RDA: A human dietary requirement is uncertain because of the body's ability to produce biotin. Daily intake of biotin is said to be between 100 mcg and 300 mcg. It is interesting that three to six times more biotin is excreted in the urine than is ingested, reflecting the major contributions of intestinal microorganisms.

Choline

Function: Choline aids in the metabolism of fat and in the normal functioning of nerves, but other dietary elements can supplement or entirely replace it. Choline is probably not a true vitamin.

Excess: No known effects.

Deficiency: Despite serious attempts, experimentally induced choline deficiency has never resulted or been produced and, thus, there should be no concern about a spontaneous deficiency.

Food sources: Choline is present in egg yolk, whole grains, wheat germ, beans, and meats of all types.

RDA: Not established. Mixed diets are estimated to provide human adults with 400 to 900 mg of choline daily.

Folacin (folic acid)

Function: Folic acid is essential for normal growth and reproduction and for the prevention of certain blood disorders. Though some animals can synthesize folic acid in the intestine, man cannot.

Excess: In high doses, folic acid can mask the presence of pernicious anemia. Folic acid is, therefore, restricted to 0.1 mg in daily vitamin supplements. Higher dosages require a prescription.

Deficiency: A deficiency results in a macrocytic anemia which resembles pernicious anemia but is without the nervous system involvement. A deficiency is not likely to occur except in chronic alcoholics.

Food sources: Richest food sources are liver, dark green leafy vegetables, nuts, whole grain cereals, and lentils.

RDA: Males and females, 11-51+ years: 400 mcg. See Table 1 for requirements for others.

Daily intakes of healthy individuals ingesting mixed diets may be as high as 2300 mcg of total folacin. However, the extent of absorption of food folacin is not known with certainty.

Niacin (nicotinic acid)

Function: Niacin is necessary for the growth and health of tissues. It also promotes appetite, proper functioning of the digestive tract, and utilization of foods.

Excess: Niacin, in high doses, causes marked dilation of the blood vessels, resulting in "flushing" of the face, increased skin temperature, and dizziness. Additionally, although the mechanism in not understood nor the long-term consequences known, it has been recently reported that large doses of this vitamin help lower serum cholesterol levels.

Deficiency: The tissues most affected by severe niacin deficiency resulting in pellagra are the skin, gastrointestinal tract, and nervous tissues. Red lesions on any skin exposed to the air and sunlight, swollen tongue, diarrhea, and mental disturbances may occur. The 3Ds—dermatitis, diarrhea, dementia—of pellagra were a common occurrence in the first third of this century.

Food sources: Liver, lean meats, whole grains, fish, nuts, yeast, and beans are high in niacin content, while milk, eggs, and cheese are low in niacin. However, the amino acid tryptophan which is present in foods such as milk and eggs can cause the body to form niacin. Therefore, the ability to acquire adequate amounts of this vitamin is greatly enhanced, and a deficiency should be unlikely to occur. However, the recent United States Health and Nutrition Survey found clinical signs of niacin deficiency, especially in blacks.

RDA: Males, 15-22 years: 20 mg. Females, 15-22 years: 14 mg. See Table 1 for requirements for others.

Pantothenic acid

Function: Pantothenic acid is essential for the metabolism of carbohydrates, fats, and proteins leading to the release of energy.

Excess: No known effects.

Deficiency: Experimentally induced deficiencies result in fatigue, nausea, and impaired coordination, but a spontaneously occurring deficiency has not definitely been reported. Some workers have reported that the vitamin relieves the "burning feet syndrome," but this condition is certainly not due solely (no pun intended) to a pantothenic acid deficiency.

Food sources: As the name implies ("derived from everywhere"), pantothenic acid exists in all cells of living tissues and it is, thus, most unlikely that a deficiency will occur. Best sources are organ meats, egg yolk, peanuts, broccoli, cauliflower, cabbage, whole grains, and cereal brans. Meat, milk, and fruits are also moderately good sources.

RDA: Insufficient evidence exists on which to base recommended allowances. Dietary intakes in the adult population of the United States range between 5 and 20 mg/day. A daily intake of 5-10 mg is probably adequate for all adults; the upper level is suggested for pregnant and nursing women.

Riboflavin (vitamin B_2)

Function: Riboflavin is essential for general health and growth and for the health of tissues of ectodermal origin, such as the skin, eyes, and nerves. Riboflavin-containing enzymes assist in the metabolism of carbohydrates, of amino acids, and of fats—a process necessary for the production of energy.

Excess: None known.

Deficiency: A riboflavin deficiency may result in cracks in the corners of the mouth and localized inflammation. Many other causes can bring about this same problem, however. Visual symptoms may occur such as abnormal vascularization, visual fatigue and "sandy" feeling, and even a sensitivity to light. Inflammation of the tongue and skin problems around the nose and genital area also may occur. Intestinal bacteria probably manufacture small amounts of riboflavin, thus preventing a serious clinical deficiency.

Food sources: Milk supplies about 43 percent of all the riboflavin consumed by Americans. If your diet contains little or no milk, you should eat liberal amounts of liver, leafy vegetables, or beans. Eggs are also a good source of this vitamin.

RDA: Males, 15-22 years: 1.8 mg. Females, 15-22 years: 1.4 mg. See Table 1 for requirements for others.

Thiamin (vitamin B_1)

Function: Thiamin plays a role in promoting appetite and proper functioning of the digestive tract, factors important in the promotion of growth.

Excess: The body has no means of storing any excess of this vitamin. Thus, no benefit derives from taking large doses; the excess is lost in the urine.

Deficiency: Thiamin is sometimes referred to as the morale vitamin because diets deficient in this vitamin can lead to fatigue, irritability, and depression. Our diets provide enought thiamin to prevent clear-cut cases of beriberi in this country, but nervous symptoms due to a lack of this vitamin are often seen in chronic alcoholics. A recent health and nutrition survey also shows others in the population to be at risk for a thiamin deficiency.

Beriberi remains a world-wide public health problem in underdeveloped countries where rice is the basic and prevalent staple. Signs and symptoms result from involvement of the cardiovascular, gastrointestinal, muscular, and nervous systems.

Food sources: Richest sources are pork, organ meats, liver sausage, beans, potatoes, and nuts. Other lean meats, green leafy vegetables, fish, eggs, and milk are fair sources.

RDA: Males, 15-22 years: 1.5 mg. Females, 15-22 years: 1.1 mg. See Table 1 for requirements for others.

Vitamin B_6 (pyridoxine)

Function: Vitamin B_6 is essential to the metabolism of protein and amino acids and, interestingly, is necessary in the formation of niacin from tryptophan mentioned elsewhere. Vitamin B_6 is involved in red blood cell regeneration and normal functioning of nervous tissues, and appears to be needed for protection against various infections and diseases.

Excess: No untoward reactions have been reported. Large doses are used to treat iron resistant hypochromic anemia due to pyridoxine deficiency.

Deficiency: Prolonged B_6 deficiency can produce serious symptoms, including convulsions, though the most common symptoms are a dermatitis, inflammation of the tongue, and diarrhea. Most diets provide an adequate amount of this vitamin to prevent a deficiency.

Food sources: The best sources of this vitamin are meats, especially liver, some vegetables, wheat germ, wheat bran, and whole grain cereals. Procesed or refined foods are very low in B_6 and thus, foods such as white bread, precooked rice, noodles, macaroni, and spaghetti are quite low in B_6 content.

RDA: Males and females, 15-51+ years: 2.0 mg. See Table 1 for requirements for others.

There is, however, some evidence that the use of oral steroid contraceptives is accompanied by the urinary loss of tryptophan metabolities. The amount of vitamin B_6 necessary to prevent or correct these changes in women taking steroid contraceptives appears to be far greater than the amount that can be supplied by diet.

Vitamin B_{12}

Function: Vitamin B_{12} is necessary for the normal functioning of all body cells, particularly those of the bone marrow, the nervous system, and the gastrointestinal tract.

Excess: No effects known.

Deficiency: Deficiencies from dietary insufficiency result in weakness, weight loss, back pain, and nervous disorders. Deficiencies resulting from a faulty absorption mechanism give rise to pernicious anemia which, if not treated, can lead to death. People who follow a pure vegetarian diet containing no milk, eggs, or other foods of animal origin run the risk of developing an anemia or, more commonly, neurological manifestations of a vitamin B_{12} deficiency. A deficiency is not likely to occur otherwise.

Appendix II—Vitamins and Minerals

Food sources: Vitamin B_{12} is unique among vitamins in that it is not found in any plants except in minute amounts which might be absorbed from the soil. Soil is one of the better sources of B_{12} because of its high bacterial content. The original source of the vitamin is probably bacterial fermentation in the intestinal tract of animals. Liver and kidney are excellent sources of B_{12}; muscle meat and fish supply moderate amounts; whole milk lesser quantities.

RDA: Males and females, 11-51+ years: 3.0 mcg. See Table 1 for requirements for others.

The "average" diet in the United States probably supplies between 5 and 15 mcg/day, but the range can be from as low as 1 mcg to as high as 100 mcg/day. Although B_{12} occurs naturally bound to protein, most of the vitamin in foods is readily available for absorption during digestion. Pure vegetarians require vitamin B_{12} supplementation.

Minerals and Trace Elements

Mineral elements can be divided into two groups: those needed in the diet at levels of 100 mg/day or more, and those needed in amounts no higher than a few milligrams per day (the "trace elements").

Of the 103 known elements, 11 constitute the bulk of living matter. Many of the remaining 92 can be detected in water, plants, and animals when sensitive methods are used. However, biological function in animals has been demonstrated, as yet, for only 17 trace elements. While all of these, and probably others, may eventually prove essential for man, there are only a few for which the present state of knowledge allows an evaluation for human nutrition.

To quote from the report on Recommended Allowances by the National Academy of Sciences:[1]

> Two trends may lead to imbalances of trace element nutrition in the future. First, increasing consumption of highly refined or fabricated foods substantially reduces the intake of essential micronutrients, unless these foods are fortified to concentrations at least equal to those naturally occurring in the products that they replace. (Meat, fish, and some nonpartitioned vegetable products are good sources of essential elements, a fact that increases their nutritional value beyond simply serving as protein sources.) Second, human exposure to environments contaminated with certain heavy metals for which no essential function is known has increased, and can be expected to increase further in the future. The consequences for health of these imbalances are little known, but trace elements, like many nutrients, can cause

injury at excessive levels of intake. In view of the highly variable distribution patterns of trace elements in foods, the consumption of varied and balanced diets is an important means whereby to avoid the extremes of deficient or excessive intake.

Calcium and phosphorus

Function: Calcium and phosphorus have a number of essential roles. The one we are all most familiar with is tooth and bone development. Ninety-nine percent of the body's calcium supply and 80 to 85 percent of the body's phosphorus supply is found in the bones. Until this day, it seems mind-boggling to realize that the skeleton of a young child is completely replaced between ages one and two years. There are two different kinds of cells which are constantly altering bone structure even in adult life. Metabolism is slower in the adult, however, and the turnover takes about 10 to 12 years. Though major bone growth is over by age 18, there still follows a period of a few years where the bone continues to become more solid.

Calcium is also necessary for the proper functioning of muscles — such as maintaining cardiac contraction — a normal pulse, and to a portion of the nervous system. It is essential for the clotting of blood. Phosphorus has more functions than any other mineral in the body. It plays an important part in almost all metabolic processes.

Excess: Unless there is an excessive intake of vitamin D — which aids in the absorption of calcium — ill effects are not likely to occur. However, excessive calcium intake should be avoided by those who have had kidney "stones" which have been shown to contain calcium. There are no known ill effects associated with large amounts of dietary phosphorus.

Deficiency: Insufficient intake of calcium and phosphorus, as well as a marked imbalance in calcium-phosphorus intake, may result in rickets in children, a disease characterized by skeletal malformations such as bowed legs, knock-knees, curvature of the spine, and pelvic and chest deformities. Tooth development is hindered and decay is prevalent. Osteomalacia, a disease characterized by a gradual softening and bending of the bones can occur in adults but this is unlikely except where pregnancy adds stress to an already malnourished body.

There is some suggestion that an inadequate calcium intake in early adult life may be one of the many factors linked to the development of osteoporosis (reduction in the quantity of bone) in middle or old age. Unfortunately, the recent health and nutrition survey done in this country showed signs of calcium-phosphorus imbalance in a large segment of our population.

Food sources: Phosphorus is present in all plants and animals; it is only when your diet contains large amounts of refined or processed foods that the phosphorus content is likely to be greatly reduced. Milk and cheese are

Appendix II—Vitamins and Minerals

the most valuable sources of calcium, though the small amount of calcium found in cereals shouldn't be overlooked because of the large amounts of cereal eaten by most Americans. Vitamin D is, however, required for efficient absorption.

Incidentally, in skimmed or low-fat milk only the fat is missing; most of the protein, vitamins, and minerals are still there. Vitamin D-fortified milk is the wisest choice as very little of this vitamin is found in natural foods.

An interesting experiment that you might like to try to show how calcium gives rigidity to bones is to take a chicken bone and let it stand in vinegar for several days. As the vinegar dissolves the calcium in the bone, the bone will become pliable. The fact that the bone does not entirely dissolve also illustrates the presence of other minerals in the bone in addition to calcium.

RDA: Males and females, 11-18 years: 1200 mg each of calcium and phosphorus. Males and Females, 19-51+ years: 800 mg each. See Table 1 for requirements for others.

Chloride

Function: Chloride, a common water purifier and bleach, is required to maintain the body's chemical balance. It also has a special function in forming hydrochloric acid which is necessary for proper absorption of vitamin B_{12} and iron.

Excess: Anything that disturbs the body's electrolyte balance is dangerous. Actually, since most of our chloride comes from our use of salt, to have an excess of chloride you would also have an excess of sodium. Therefore, the precautions noted for sodium would also apply here.

Deficiency: Loss of chloride generally parallels that of sodium, and a separate deficiency occurs only when there is loss of chloride due to vomiting. Symptoms include nausea, diarrhea, and abdominal and muscular cramps.

Food sources: Most of our supply of chloride comes from our use of salt which is a combination of sodium and chloride. Our daily diet supplies chloride far in excess of bodily needs, so there is no reason to try and supplement your supply.

RDA: Not established.

Chromium

Function: Chromium has a variety of functions, including: 1) stimulation of enzymes involved in glucose and energy metabolism; 2) stimulation of the synthesis of fatty acids and cholesterol in the liver; 3) involvement in insulin metabolism; and 4) a role as a part of several other enzymes including one of protein-digesting enzymes in the intestine.

Excess: Not known.

Deficiency: Poorly nourished children in several parts of the Middle East where chromium levels of some soils and water supplies appear to be low, show signs of poor glucose utilization. This has been explained on the basis of the role of chromium in insulin metabolism. Similar effects have been seen in a few diabetic adults who apparently were deficient in chromium. Recent indications that chromium may play a role in the prevention of atherosclerosis in man and cholesterol metabolism in animals have not been confirmed.

Food sources: Most animal (except fish) proteins, whole grain products, and brewer's yeast are good sources of available chromium.

RDA: In view of the greatly varying availability of chromium in different foods, a meaningful recommendation for chromium intake cannot be given as yet. The average daily loss, mainly through the urine, is 7-10 mcg.

Cobalt

Function: Cobalt is an essential structural part of the vitamin B_{12} molecule. There is no evidence that this element has a function in the normal nutrition of man other than as a part of vitamin B_{12}.

Excess: Undue amounts of cobalt in the diet of man and animal species other than ruminants cause stimulation of bone marrow, with excessive production of red corpuscles and higher than normal hemoglobin. An outbreak of cardiomyopathy in Canada may have been due to cobalt deliberately added to beer to improve its "head."

Deficiency: A cobalt deficiency has never been described for man.

Food sources: Cobalt is present in almost all foods in varying amounts.

RDA: Not established.

Copper

Function: Copper is necessary for melanin pigment formation in the body, and aids in the absorption and use of iron in the synthesis of hemoglobin and in the absorption of vitamin C. It is also necessary for the metabolism of glucose and the release of energy, the protection of the nervous system, and the formation of connective tissue.

Excess: Since copper cooking utensils are rarely used now, there is little danger of toxicity occuring. In high concentrations, however, copper is definitely poisonous.

Deficiency: There is no evidence of a dietary deficiency of copper ever occurring in man. Even the poorest of foods contain copper and the human diet provides more than enough copper. Death from caloric starvation would probably occur before any clear clinical sign of a deficiency would appear. Actually, natural drinking water often supplies the body's entire requirement.

Food sources: Richest sources are organ meats, shellfish, nuts, beans, cocoa, and whole grain cereals.

Appendix II—Vitamins and Minerals

RDA: Not established. Copper intakes of 1.3 and 2.0 mg/day appear to maintain balance in preadolescent girls and adults, respectively. The requirement of infants and children has been estimated at between 0.05 and 0.1 mg/kg of body weight per day; an intake of 0.08 mg/kg/day appears to be adequate.

Women taking contraceptive medication and patients with certain infectious diseases have been found to have elevated serum copper concentrations, but the nutritional implications of these findings have not been clearly established. A metabolic condition (Wilson's disease) requires a drastic reduction of copper-rich foods.

Fluorine

Function: Fluorine is of great importance to the development of teeth resistant to decay. This element is deposited in the enamel surface of the developing teeth of children. It is not deposited in fully developed adult teeth; thus, adults exposed to adequate fluorine intake for the first time cannot expect any such benefit. Additionally, there is some suggestion that moderate amounts in the bone may reduce osteoporosis (a decalcification of the bone). Therefore, it is possible that fluorinated water may be beneficial for the geriatric generation's bones, if not for their teeth.

Excess: "Mottling" of the teeth. This condition is seen in communities where the natural water supply contains from 2 to 6 ppm of fluroine—for example, Colorado and the Texas panhandle. Artificial fluorination of water supplies is usually at about the 1 ppm level, which will not cause mottling. Fluorine, like other trace elements, is toxic when consumed in excessive amounts. However, the daily intakes required to produce symptoms of chronic toxicity after years of consumption are 20 to 80 mg or more, far in excess of the average intake in the United States.

Deficiency: Increased incidence of tooth decay. Some studies have suggested a possible function of fluorine is the maintenance of bone structure, but further investigation of this point is required.

Food sources: Most of our supply of fluorine comes from our drinking water. Fluorine is naturally present in hard water, but it has also become a widespread practice in this country to artificially fluorinate drinking water. Opposition to this addition of fluorine is ususally based on faulty information about the amount of this element that is tolerable by man. Other significant sources of fluorine are sea-fish and tea, especially China tea. Fluorine is present in small but widely varying concentrations in practically all soils, water supplies, plants, and animals.

RDA: Not established.

Iodine

Function: Iodine is heavily concentrated in the thyroid gland and is a part of the hormones secreted by that gland. As these secretions determine the level of metabolism in many cells and also play a part in the control of connective tissue, the importance of this element is evident.

Excess: Large doses taken over a long period of time can depress thyroid function.

Deficiency: The most well-known condition resulting from iodine deficiency is goitre, an enlargement of the thyroid gland. The use of iodized salt in the United States makes a deficiency unlikely unless one's diet is severely salt-restricted during pregnancy, a time when one's need for iodine is inincreased. The mental retardation in congenital cretinism, caused by the fetus receiving an inadequate supply of iodine, is irreversible unless the condition is recognized immediately after birth and thyroid therapy started early. It can be seen, thus, that both the mother and the child stand to suffer if an iodine deficiency occurs during pregnancy.

Food sources: The iodine content of plants and animals is determined by the environment in which they grow. As most soils contain little iodine, most foodstuffs are poor sources. The only rich source of iodine is seafood. Most of our iodine comes through the use of iodized salt. However, only slightly more than half of the table salt consumed in the United States is iodized, so check the label. Salt added to preprocessed foods by the manufacturer usually does not contain iodine, and salt bought in bulk—for example, by schools and restaurant chains—is unlikely to be iodized. It is recommended that only iodized salt be used in the household.

It should be remembered that even though iodization programs have proven successful as preventive measures, increased iodine intake is unlikely to reduce the size of the thyroid gland once goitre has developed. It is of concern that the recent health and nutrition survey showed evidence of iodine deficiency, especially in black women of ages 18 to 44 and black youths age 12 to 17.

RDA: Males, 11-51+ years: varies between 110 and 130 mcg. Females, 11-51+ years: varies between 80 and 115 mcg. See Table 1 for details as well as requirements for others.

Iron

Function: Iron is utilized primarily by bone marrow to make red blood cells and to prevent anemia. Since the life of these cells is only about 120 days, you can see why it is critical to maintain an adequate iron intake; this is especially true for women because of blood losses during menstruation.

Excess: Detrimental to unfortunate rare individuals with a chronic iron storage disease throughout the body called hemochromatosis. Also, can prove fatal when taken in large doses. The average human lethal dose is about 200 to 250 mg of iron per kilogram of body weight. Lethargy, vomiting (without

Appendix II—Vitamins and Minerals

or with blood—caustic effect), fast and weak pulse, low blood pressure, pallor, cyanosis, ataxia, and coma may appear within one-half to one hour after ingestion. These symptoms may disappear after four to six hours, followed by a 6- to 24-hour period in which the individual seems to improve rapidly. A second crisis may then occur with cyanosis, vasomotor collapse, pulmonary edema, coma, and death within 12 to 48 hours.

Deficiency: A deficient supply of iron is a common cause of a mild anemia with resultant loss of vitality. During the reproductive period of a woman's life, losses of iron are inevitable. These occur at the time of menstrual periods, and in pregnancy with the transfer of iron to her infant, first when it is in the uterus and later when nursing. Thus, a woman during these years has a loss of iron at least double that of a man or a woman after the menopause. This should not lure males into a false sense of security, however. A recent nutritional survey done in the United States showed that 95 percent of all preschool children—male and female—have iron intakes below standard. Actually, males aged 18 to 44 years were the only group that showed adequate iron intakes.

As a result of the United States survey, the Food and Drug Administration has proposed increasing the amount of iron added to flour and bread in this country. This proposal is opposed by some medical and lay groups, however. Their feeling is that: the number of states and the segments of the population included in the survey are not an adequate sample and should not be construed as representative of this nation as a whole; dietary intakes are not necessarily adequate indicators of individual nutritional status; and adequate proof is lacking of either the effectiveness of this proposal in preventing iron deficiency anemia or the safety of the proposed measure. Additionally, there is concern that this proposed addition of iron might be hazardous to people who suffer from iron-storage diseases such as hemochromatosis and thalasemia.

Obviously, there is much that still isn't known about diet evaluation and the effects of certain deficiencies and excesses!

Food sources: Liver is one of the richest sources of iron. Luckily, the very green leafy vegetables are also a fairly good source, as are some beans. Milk is a poor source of iron, which is the reason for the use of iron-enriched milks and cereals, egg yolk, meat, and green leafy vegetables in infant feeding. Pumpkin seeds are also a good source of iron.

RDA: Males, 11-51+ years: varies between 10 and 18 mg. Females, 11-50 years: 18 mg. See Table 1 for details and for requirements for others.

Magnesium

Function: Magnesium is an essential part of many complex functions required for the release of energy. It is a component of soft tissues as well as bone. Cardiac and skeletal muscle and nervous tissue depend on a proper balance between calcium and magnesium for normal function.

Excess: No known effects from food sources. Certain disease conditions such as renal failure and Addison's disease, and misuse of magnesium sulfate can produce depression of respiration, deep tendon reflexes, drowsiness, and coma. These symptoms are rapidly reversed by IV administration of calcium.

Deficiency: A true dietary deficiency has not been reported. Deficiency has only been noted as a result of a disease process, such as renal disease, toxemia of pregnancy, or chronic alcoholism with hepatic cirrhosis.

Food sources: Most foods, especially vegetables, contain useful amounts of magnesium and it is, therefore, unlikely that magnesium deficiency will arise unless there is chronic diarrhea present.

RDA: Males, 11-51+ years: 350-400 mg. Females, 11-51+ years: 300 mg. See Table 1 for details and for requirements for others.

Manganese

Function: Manganese is an important catalyst and is a part of many enzymes in the body. On the basis of its relationship to these enzymes, it is needed for many functions, including the synthesis of complex carbohydrates. Few elements have as many metabolic functions as does manganese.

Excess: Manganese poisoning occurs in workers at manganese mines. The signs and symptoms are those of a generalized disease of the central nervous system. Otherwise, this element is relatively nontoxic.

Deficiency: Manganese deficiency has not been reported in man, but can be produced in many laboratory animals and may occur in cattle grazing on peat pastures, which are poor in manganese.

Food sources: Manganese is widely distributed in foods of plant and animal origin, though it is lost along with other trace elements in food refining. Cereals, peas, beans, lentils, nuts, and especially tea and coffee are the main sources.

RDA: Not established. The average daily intake is estimated to be 2.5 to 7.0 mg.

Molybdenum

Function: Molybdenum is a component of at least one essential enzyme. A catalytic role in fatty acid oxidation has also been attributed to molybdenum.

Excess: Unknown but unlikely.

Deficiency: Deficiencies have been produced in animals, but are unknown in man.

Food sources: The molybdenum content of foods varies greatly; beef kidney, some but not all cereals, and some legumes appear to be good sources.

Appendix II—Vitamins and Minerals

RDA: Not established. The estimated daily intake in the United States is 45 to 500 mcg.

Nickel

Function: Nickel's close similarity to cobalt in chemical properties suggests that it might have some essential enzymic property in animal tissues. Little is known of its need by man.

Excess: Unknown but unlikely.

Deficiency: Deficiency has been produced in experimental animals, but has never been seen in man.

Food sources: Nickel is widely distributed in foods, especially plant foods.

RDA: Not established.

Potassium

Function: Like sodium and chloride, potassium is also required to maintain the electrolyte balance of the body.

Excess: Excesses are usually seen as a complication of medical treatment of other conditions. Excesses can result in serious cardiac irregularities, which can progress to cardiac arrest.

Deficiency: Potassium deficiency is a factor in diabetic coma. It can also occur with prolonged diarrhea, abnormal kidney function, and renal disease. Potassium deficiency is manifested by muscular weakness, increased nervous irritability, mental disorientation, and cardiac irregularities. It is unlikely that potassium deficiency or excess will occur as a result of dietary intake for the average person.

Food sources: Most foods, especially citrus fruits, contain potassium but in widely varying amounts. You do not need to work at maintaining your potassium level; it sort of takes care of itself.

RDA: Not established. It is estimated that healthy adults need about 2.5 grams per day.

Selenium

Function: Selenium is in all probability required by humans, just as it is for experimental animal studies thus far. However, final experimental proof of its need for man has not yet been obtained.

Excess: Animals grazing in areas with toxic levels of selenium developed symptoms of "alkali disease" or "blind staggers" characterized by stiffness and lameness, loss of hair, deformed hoofs, blindness, paralysis, and eventually death. Toxic symptoms in man are somewhat similar, but also include an increased incidence of dental caries.

Deficiency: Very little is known about the human requirement for selenium. A wide variety of symptoms can be seen in selenium-deficient animals.

Food sources: Selenium, probably bound to protein, occurs naturally in all seafood, meat, and those grains raised on selenium-containing soils. Considerable losses can occur in processing, refinement of foods, and cooking.

RDA: Not established. A person eating a mixed diet of foods of different origins would most likely be getting about 50 to 100 mcg of selenium per day. This amount appears to be more than the amount needed.

Silicon

Function: Silicon has long been known to be required by certain forms of life and, apparently, some plants, but its need by animals for growth and bone development was only recently discovered.

Excess: Unknown but unlikely.

Deficiency: Poor growth in animals.

Food sources: Silicon is widely distributed in foods. On the basis of present knowledge, a deficiency in man seems virtually impossible.

RDA: Not established.

Sodium

Function: Sodium is necessary in maintaining the body's fluid balance, which is crucial to the body's well-being.

Excess: There is increasing evidence that intakes of salt—salt is approximately 40 percent sodium and 60 percent chloride—beyond physiological requirements are harmful to your health. For example, where salt intake is consistently high, as in Japan, there is an increased incidence of high blood pressure. Other studies have shown that people who salt their food without tasting it first are more likely to suffer from high blood pressure than those who taste first then salt, while the latter group is more at risk than those who never salt at all. Additionally, excessive amounts of sodium cause the body to retain unusual amounts of water in an attempt to bring the body into chemical balance. The result is increased weight and edema (swelling). This can be harmful to the kidneys and to the lungs.

Deficiency: Sodium deficiency can be described as a state where the amounts of sodium and body fluids are not in balance. This imbalance can result from a loss of sodium through the skin in excessive overheating and consequent sweating, or by the intake of too much water without accompanying sodium—usually in response to great thirst after excessive sweating. The usual symptoms of this imbalance are muscular cramping and weakness, though if the sodium depletion or water intoxication is severe enough, loss of consciousness and even convulsions can occur. The possibility of such an imbalance is of especial concern to athletes.

Food sources: We hasten to say that under normal circumstances you do not need to purposely add sodium to your diet. Though most foods are low in

sodium content, large amounts are often added in processing or preserving by the addition of salt.
RDA: Not established.

Sulfur

Function: All living matter contains proteins and all proteins contain some sulfur. This element is, therefore, essential for life. It is important to the functioning of some enzyme systems.

Excess: Not well documented.

Deficiency: Little is known of sulfur requirements or sulfur deficiency in man.

Food sources: It is likely that most of the required sulfur is obtained through the amino acids menthionine and cystine, plus the vitamins thiamin and biotin. Sulfur is found in eggs, meat, milk, cheese, nuts, and legumes. Onions are a particularly rich source of organic sulfur.

RDA: Not established.

Tin

Function: Tin has an important growth-promoting effect in animals. No studies showing a requirement for tin by man have been made as yet, but the results with rats suggest its need.

Excess: Tin is not very toxic, though gastrointestinal irritation can occur when acid fruit juices or similar products dissolve appreciable amounts of tin from a tin-plated can.

Deficiency: A reduced growth-rate can be produced in animals.

Food sources: Tin is widely distributed in foods of plant and animal origin, and a deficiency in man or animals under normal conditions would not be expected to occur.

RDA: Not established.

Vanadium

Function: Vanadium is known to be a catalyst in several biological systems and to be present in higher than normal concentrations in teeth.

Excess: Unknown but unlikely. Ascorbic acid (vitamin C) has been found to be an effective antidote for poisoning in animals.

Deficiency: Poor growth in animals.

Food sources: Vanadium is present throughout the plant and animal kingdoms.

RDA: Not established. No figure can be given for the vanadium requirement of man, but it would appear to be in the range of only 0.1 to 0.3 mg per day. Normal diets contain about ten times this amount.

Zinc

Function: Zinc is essential for normal growth of the genital organs, prevention of anemia, general growth of all tissues, and wound healing.

Excess: Poisoning has been known to occur from drinking acid fruit drinks that had been stored in galvanized containers.

Deficiency: Zinc is widely distributed in foods, and a deficiency is most unlikely to occur, except in diets limited to vegetable sources of protein. However, in Iranian men the excessive consumption of wheat containing large amounts of phosphate which inhibits zinc and iron absorption has produced severe anemia, dermatitis, and dwarfism. All symptoms responded to zinc therapy except for the anemia which required iron.

Food Sources: Oysters are an unusually rich source, whereas plant foods are a generally poor source. Zinc is also found in organ meats and seafood.

RDA: Males and females, 11-51+ years: 15 mg. See Table 1 for requirements for others. The average zinc content of a mixed diet consumed by the American adult is between 10 and 15 mg.

Nonessential Trace Elements (for Higher Animals)

Many other trace elements are known to be present in plants and animals. Any of these could conceivably be shown to be essential in the diet of man at some time in the future. There are small pieces of evidence for a possible future role in nutrition for some, such as boron. There are other elements such as gold, antimony, cesium, lead, lithium, and mercury which are widely distributed in nature but which do not appear to have any biological function. However, it is well to remember that tin, nickel, selenium, chromium, silicon, vanadium, and cadmium were listed with these nonessential elements just a few years ago!

Notes

Food, Glorious Food
1. *Recommended Dietary Allowances,* Food and Nutrition Board, National Academy of Sciences (Washington: National Academy of Sciences, 1974), p.10

Food for Thought
1. Lawrence E. Lamb, M.D., *What You Need to Know About Food & Cooking for Health* (New York: Viking Press, 1973), p. 272.

At the Store and In Your Kitchen
1. *American Heart Association Cookbook* (New York: David McKay Company, Inc. 1973), pp. xxiii-xxxiv. Copyright 1973 and 1975 by The American Heart Association. Reprinted by permission of the publisher.

Special Dietary Problems
1. Sir Stanley Davidson, R. Passmore, and J.F. Brock, *Human Nutrition and Dietetics* (Baltimore: Williams & Wilkins Company, 1972), p. 509.

Appendix II
1. *Recommended Dietary Allowances,* p. 91-92.

Bibliography

Abiaka, M. H. "Japanese-American Food Equivalents for Calculating Exchange Diets." *J. Am. Diet. Assn.* 62:173-180, Feb. 1973.

American Association for Health, Physical Education, and Recreation. *Nutrition for Athletes. A Handbook for Coaches.* Washington, D.C.: Amer. Assn. for Health, Physical Education, and Recreation, 1971.

American Dietetic Association. *Food Facts Talk Back.* Chicago: The American Dietetic Assn. (undated).

American Heart Association. *The American Heart Association Cookbook.* New York: David McKay, 1973.

Ames Company. *Toward Good Control. A Guidebook for the Diabetic.* Indiana: Ames Co.-Miles Laboratories, 1973.

Arona, J.M *Poisoning. Toxicology-Symptoms-Treatments.* Illinois: Chas. C. Thomas, 1974.

Bogert, L.J.; Briggs, G.M.; and Calloway, D.H. *Nutrition and Physical Fitness.* Philadelphia: W.B. Saunders Co., 1973.

Bray, G.A., and Bethune, J.E. *Treatment and Management of Obesity.* New York: Harper & Row, 1974.

Burton, B.T. *The Heinz Handbook of Nutrition. A Comprehensive Treatise on Nutrition in Health and Disease.* New York: McGraw-Hill, 1965.

Carson, R. *Silent Spring.* New York: Fawcett World Library, 1964.

Christakis, G., and Plumb, R.K. *Obesity.* New York: The Nutrition Foundation, 1966.

Church, C.F., and Church, H.N. *Food Values of Portions Commonly Used.* Philadelphia: J.B. Lippincott, 1970.

Consumer Reports. "Acne Remedies. Clearing Up the Confusion." February

1974, pgs. 151-153.

Coulehan, J.L., et al. "Vitamin C Prophylaxis in a Boarding School." *NE J Med* 290, no. 1:6-10, Jan. 3, 1974.

Craddock, D. *Obesity and its Management.* London: Churchill Livingstone, 1973.

Crosby, W.H. "Can a Vegetarian be Well Nourished?" *JAMA* 233, no. 8: 898, Aug. 25, 1975.

Crosby, W.H. "Mercury in Fish." *JAMA* 233, no.9:1001-1002, Sept. 1, 1975.

Dack, G.M. *Food Poisoning.* Chicago: University of Chicago Press, 1956.

Davidson, S.S.; Passmore, R.; and Brock, J.F. *Human Nutrition and Dietetics.* Baltimore: Williams & Wilkins, 1972.

Dawber, T.R.; Kannel, W.B.; and Gordon, T. "Coffee and Cardiovascular Disease." *NE J Med* 291, no. 17:871-877, Oct. 24, 1974.

DHEW Publication No. (HRA)74-1219-1. *Preliminary Findings of the First Health and Nutrition Examination Survey, United States, 1971-1972. Dietary Intake and Biochemical Findings.* Maryland: National Center for Health Statistics, Jan. 1974.

DHEW Publication No. (HRA) 75-1229. *Preliminary Findings of the First Health and Nutrition Examination Survey, United States, 1971-72. Anthropometric and Clinical Findings.* Maryland: National Center for Health Statistics, 1975.

Erhard, D. The New Vegetarians. "Part One-Vegetarianism and its Medical Consequences." *Nutrition Today,* Nov./Dec. 1973, pgs. 4-12.

Federal Register. *Label Statements Concerning Dietary Properties of Food Purporting to be or Represented for Special Dietary Uses.* Vol. 38:20717, Aug. 2, 1973.

Food and Nutrition Board, National Research Council. *Recommended Dietary Allowances.* Washington, D.C.: National Academy of Sciences, 1974.

Geigy Pharmaceuticals. *Documenta Geigy. Scientific Tables.* Ardsley, New York: Geigy Pharmaceuticals, 1970.

Gifft, H.H.; Washbon, M.B.; and Harrison, G.G. *Nutrition, Behavior, and Change.* New Jersey: Prentice-Hall, 1972.

Hardin, J.W. and Arena, J.M. *Human Poisoning from Native and Cultivated Plants.* Durham, N.C.: Duke University Press, 1974.

Herbert, V., and Jacob E. "Destruction of Vitamin B^{12} by Ascorbic Acid." *JAMA* 230, no. 2:241-242, Oct. 14, 1974.

Jones, J. *The Calculating Cook.* San Francisco: 101 Productions, 1972.

Lamb, L.E. *What You Need to Know about Food and Cooking for Health.* New York: Viking Press, 1973.

Mayer, J. *Overweight. Causes, Cost, and Control.* New Jersey: Prentice-Hall, 1968.

Medical World News. "Dealing with Food Poisoning." Aug. 25, 1975, pgs. 74-83.

Medical World News. "More Iron in Bread—Who Needs It?" April 19, 1974, pgs. 27-28.

North Carolina Dietetic Association, Inc. *Diet Manual.* North Carolina: North Carolina Dietetic Assn., Inc., 1975.

Parker, B.C. "The Case for Conservation in Antarctica." *Antartic J of the United States* VI, no. 3, May/June, 1971.

Pimentel, D., et al. "Energy and Land Constraints in Food Protein Production." *Science* 190:754-761, November 21, 1975.

Register, U.D., and Sonnenberg, L.M. "The Vegetarian Diet." *J Am Diet Assn* 62:253-261, March 1973.

Rivlin, R.S. "Drug Therapy. Treatment of Obesity with Hormones." *NE J MED* 292, no. 1:26-29, Jan. 2, 1975.

Sacks, F.M., et al. "Plasma Lipids and Lipoproteins in Vegetarians and Controls." *NE J Med* 292, no. 22:1148-1151, May 29, 1975.

Sandoz Pharmaceuticals. *The Obese Patient.* New Jersey: Sandoz Pharmaceuticals, 1974.

Seventh-day Adventist Dietetic Association. *Diet Manual Utilizing a Vegetarian Diet Plan.* California: The Seventh-day Adventist Dietetic Assn., 1975.

Shalita, A.R. "Acne Vulgaris. Not Curable but Treatable." *Modern Medicine*: 66-76, Aug. 1, 1975.

Stare, F.J. (ed). *Atherosclerosis.* New York: MEDCOM, 1974.

Stare, F.J. (ed). *Obesity.* New York: MEDCOM, 1974.

Stuart, R.B. and Davis, B. *Slim Chance in a Fat World. Behavioral Control of Obesity.* Illinois: Research Press, 1974.

Today's Health. "Protein Supplements." June 1975, pg. 12.

Today's Health. "Tips to Prevent Food Poisoning." September, 1975, pg. 11.

Turner, J.S. *The Chemical Feast.* New York: Grossman Publishers, 1970.

US Department of Agriculture. Home and Garden Bulletin No. 72. *Nutritive Value of Foods.* Washington: US Government Printing Office, 1971.

Verrett, J. and Carper, J. *Eating May be Hazardous to Your Health.* New York: Doubleday, 1975.

Vital Health Statistics, Series 21, no. 23. *Teenagers: Marriages, Divorces, Parenthood, and Mortality.* Washington, D.C.: U.S. Government Printing Office. August 1973.

White, P.L. and Selvey, N. (eds). *Let's Talk About Food. Answers to Your Questions about Foods and Nutrition.* Massachusetts: Publishing Sciences Group, 1974.

HEALTH AND FITNESS

By Dr. Per-Olof Åstrand, the noted Swedish authority on physical fitness, who explains clearly how our bodies respond to exercise.

Advice on how to lose weight and get into shape. Training programs for home use, for those in good physical condition, and for inactive or elderly persons.

Over 90 photographs plus illustrated charts and diagrams, easy-to-remember Fit Tips, Fit Facts, and Facts on Food. $3.95

At your local bookseller or order direct adding 10% postage plus applicable sales tax.
BARRON'S, 113 Crossways Pk. Dr., Woodbury, N.Y. 11797

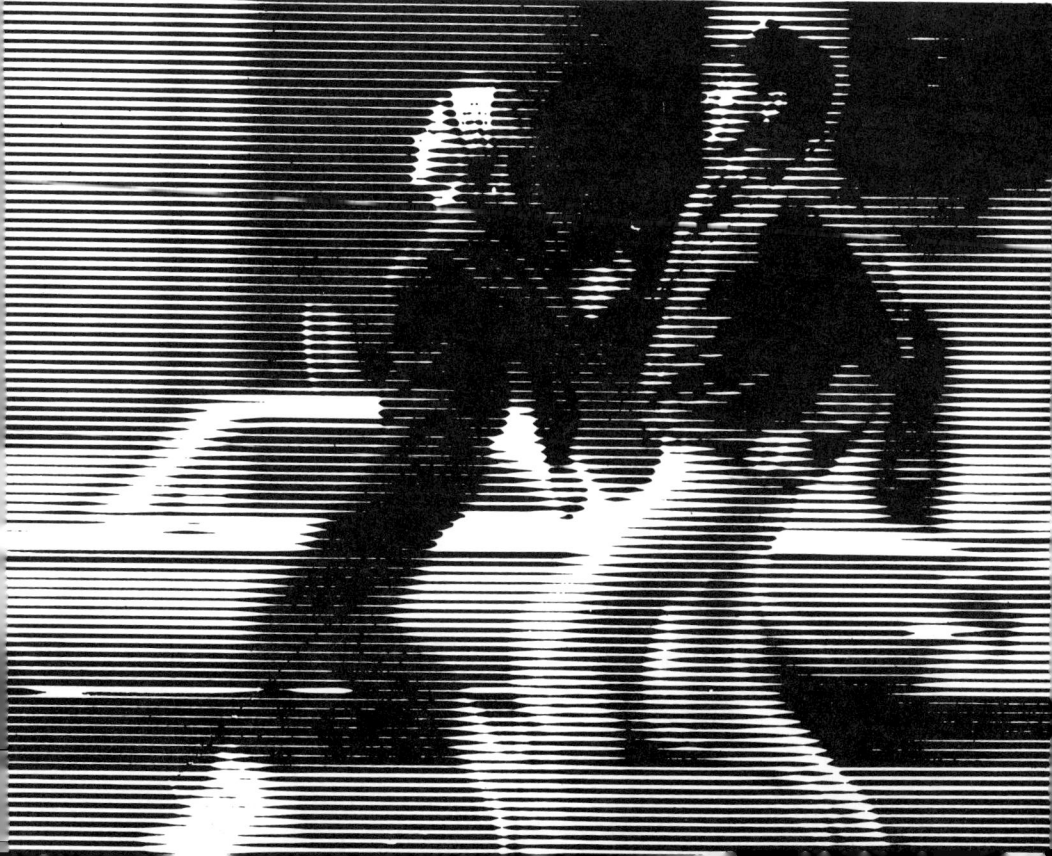

THE NATIVE ORCHIDS OF THE UNITED STATES AND CANADA EXCLUDING FLORIDA

Carlyle A. Luer

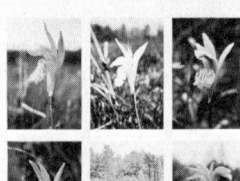

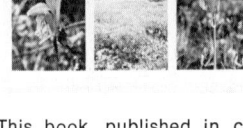

This book, published in conjunction with the New York Botanical Garden, has hundreds of color plates, diagrams, and descriptions that make it a valuable reference to all orchid species. It includes shaded maps to indicate the type of environment and the area where each flower is grown. $44.95

THE NATIVE ORCHIDS OF FLORIDA

Carlyle A. Luer

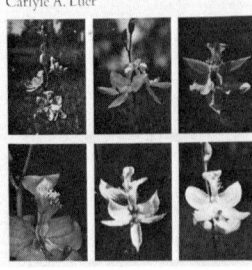

Also published with the New York Botanical Garden, this large and lovely book gives detailed descriptions as well as photographs and shaded maps of these exotic flowers native to Florida. Detailed diagrams and information on size, shape and climate requirements complete this reference book.
$39.95

WILDFLOWERS OF THE NORTHEASTERN UNITED STATES

NEW YORK BOTANICAL GARDEN'S HANDBOOK

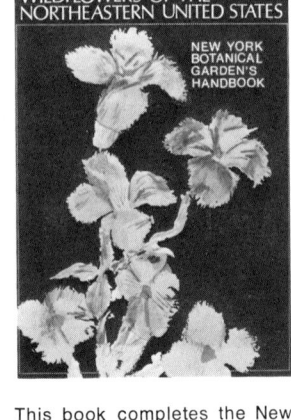

This book completes the New York Botanical Garden series, and like its companions, it provides much information on the wildflowers of the northeast. One-hundred-and-fifty color plates make this a beautiful and appealing book that is an invaluable field guide to these common flowers. $6.95

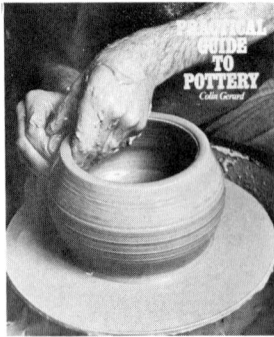

With photographs of ancient and modern pottery, instructions on types of clay, glazes, methods, and uses, this book is a comprehensive source book to the potter's craft. It is nicely balanced between historical information on pottery and information on techniques for creating distinctive works of art. $8.95

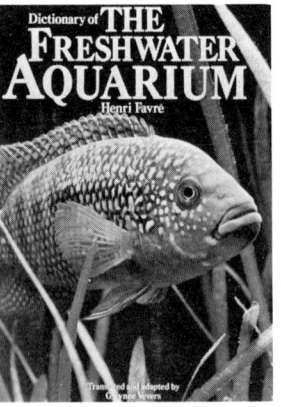

Over 180 color photographs make this an exceptional sourcebook to tropical and common freshwater aquarium fish. Presented in alphabetical encyclopedic form, it includes information on equipment, plants, food, propagation, compatability and more. With extensive cross-referencing.
$12.95

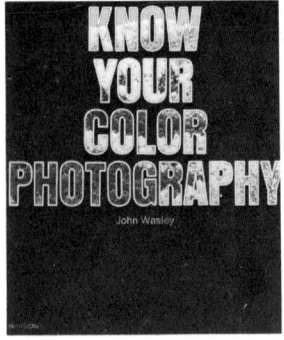

A readable basic reference for camera enthusiasts of all ages, this book covers more than technique in both color and black and white photography. Sample photographs reinforce the ideas expressed in this book and diagrams and illustrations make this an easy-to-follow guide to this ageless craft. $7.95

At your local bookseller or use coupon on following page.

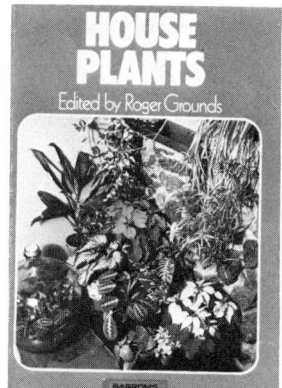

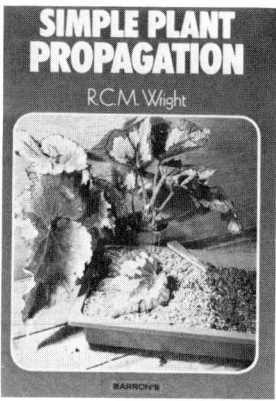

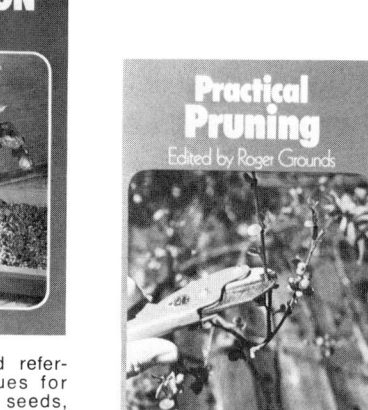

An introduction to gardening with house plants featuring hints on care and cultivation, common pests and diseases, and propagation. With specific information on individual species of foliage and flowering plants including light, temperature, and moisture requirements of each. $2.95

This heavily illustrated reference shows techniques for growing plants from seeds, dividing mature plants, working with bulbs and corms, making cuttings, grafting, and layering. Also includes information on propagating flowers, trees, and shrubs plus information on raising vegetables and herbs. $2.95

An illustrated guide to proper pruning techniques that explains what varieties need pruning, when to prune, and how to do it. With information on shrubs, roses, fruit trees, bushes, and hedges. $2.95

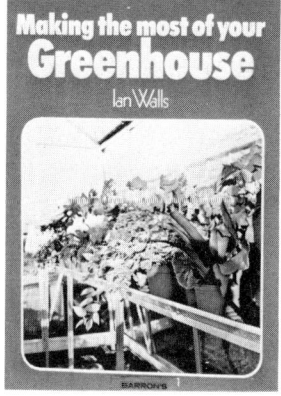

The purpose of this book is to show ways of getting the best out of your own greenhouse by making the most of the ingenious modern devices available to help run it. The range of equipment is discussed in plain language enabling the reader to grow bigger and better crops over a longer period of the year. $2.95

OTHER BOOKS IN THE SERIES

SIMPLE FRUIT GROWING

GROWING A GREEN THUMB, A picture book for children ranging from planting seeds in containers, growing vegetables and flowers, identifying garden enemies, and building a toad house to using produce.

BARRON'S 113 Crossways Park Drive, Woodbury, New York 11797

Please send me the following quantities as indicated:

_____ COMMON WILDFLOWERS OF THE NORTHEAST; (#937) $6.95 paper
_____ GROWING A GREEN THUMB; (#736) $1.95 paper
_____ HOUSE PLANTS; (#796) $2.95 paper
_____ KNOW YOUR COLOR PHOTOGRAPHY; (#5128) $7.95 cloth
_____ LAROUSSE DICTIONARY OF THE FRESH-WATER AQUARIUM; (#5192) $12.95 cloth
_____ MAKING THE MOST OF YOUR GREENHOUSE; (#869) $2.95 paper
_____ NATIVE ORCHIDS OF FLORIDA; (#5183) $39.95 cloth
_____ NATIVE ORCHIDS OF THE UNITED STATES AND CANADA EXCLUDING FLORIDA; (#5184) $44.95 cloth

_____ PRACTICAL GUIDE TO POTTERY; (#5187) $8.95 hardbound
_____ PRACTICAL PRUNING; (#797) $2.95 paper
_____ SIMPLE FRUIT GROWING; (#908) $2.95 paper
_____ SIMPLE PLANT PROPAGATION; (#795) $2.95 paper

I am enclosing a check for $_____ which includes applicable sales tax plus 8% transportation charges. Prices subject to change without notice.

Name: _____

Address: _____

City: _____ State: _____ Zip: _____

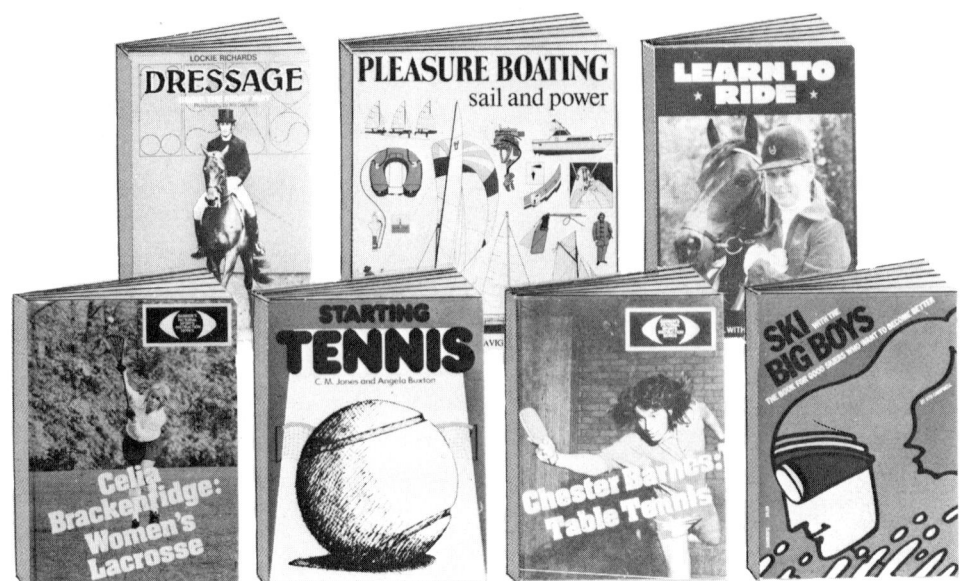

DRESSAGE: BEGIN THE RIGHT WAY
Lockie Richards; $8.95 hardbound
An instructional book filled with demonstration photos teaching the finer points of the balance and movement of horse and rider.

PLEASURE BOATING
12 international boating experts; $29.95 clothbound
A handsome, colorful volume that takes in all aspects of boating, including boat construction, safety, and navigation.

LEARN TO RIDE
Ella Winblad von Walter; $6.95 paperback, $8.95 clothbound
Step-by-step color photographs take beginners from their first encounter with a horse to the horse show.

WOMEN'S LACROSSE
Celia Brackenridge; $4.95 hardbound
Descriptions of game skills in the context of an actual game. Illustrated.

SKI WITH THE BIG BOYS
Stu Campbell; $5.95 paperback
For people who already have the basics of skiing, this book goes on to more advanced skiing techniques. Illustrated.

STARTING TENNIS
C. M. Jones and Angela Buxton; $5.95 hardbound Illustrated.
Two internationally known coaches offer beginners innovative instruction.

TABLE TENNIS
Chester Barnes; $4.95 hardbound
A pictorial sports instruction manual that explains the techniques as this international champion has come to understand them.

At your local bookseller or use coupon below.

BARRON'S   113 Crossways Park Drive, Woodbury, New York 11797
Please send me the following quantities as indicated:

____ DRESSAGE: BEGIN THE RIGHT WAY; (#5230) $8.95 cloth
____ LEARN TO RIDE; (#068) ☐ $6.95 paper, (#5112) ☐ $8.95 cloth
____ PLEASURE BOATING; (#5131) $29.95 cloth
____ SKI WITH THE BIG BOYS: (#975) $5.95 paper
____ STARTING TENNIS; (#5151) $5.95 hardbound
____ TABLE TENNIS; (#5149) $4.95 hardbound
____ WOMEN'S LACROSSE; (#5152) $4.95 hardbound

I am enclosing a check for $_____ which includes applicable sales tax plus 8% transportation. Prices subject to change without notice.

Name: _____
Address: _____
City: _____ State: _____ Zip: _____